TAKE CHARGE OF YOUR

THYROID DISORDER

Dr. Alan Christianson
& Hy Bender

ALPHA

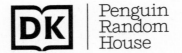

Publisher: Mike Sanders
Senior Acquisitions Editor: Janette Lynn
Copy Editor: Rick Kughen
Cover: Lindsay Dobbs
Book Designer: William Thomas
Compositor: Ayanna Lacey
Proofreader: Penny Stuart
Indexer: Celia McCoy

Alan dedicates this book to Kirin, Celestina, and Ryan.

Hy dedicates this book to you, the reader, and to your living long and joyfully with optimal health.

First American Edition, 2020
Published in the United States by DK Publishing
6081 E. 82nd Street, Indianapolis, Indiana 46250

Copyright © 2020 by Dr. Alan Christianson and Hy Bender
22 21 20   10 9 8 7 6 5 4 3 2 1
001-317281-DEC2020

Published in the United States by Dorling Kindersley Limited.

International Standard Book Number: 978-1-46549-2-678
Library of Congress Catalog Card Number: 2020931154

Interpretation of the printing code: The rightmost number of the first series of numbers is the year of the book's printing; the rightmost number of the second series of numbers is the number of the book's printing. For example, a printing code of 20-1 shows that the first printing occurred in 2020.

Printed in the United States of America

Note: This publication contains the opinions and ideas of its authors. It is intended to provide helpful and informative material on the subject matter covered. It is sold with the understanding that the authors, book producer, and publisher are not engaged in rendering professional services in the book. If the reader requires personal assistance or advice, a competent professional should be consulted.

The authors, book producer, and publisher specifically disclaim any responsibility for any liability, loss, or risk, personal or otherwise, which is incurred as a consequence, directly or indirectly, of the use and application of any of the contents of this book.

Most Alpha books are available at special quantity discounts for bulk purchases for sales promotions, premiums, fund-raising, or educational use. Special books, or book excerpts, can also be created to fit specific needs.

For details, write: Special Markets, Alpha Books, 1745 Broadway, New York, NY 10019.

Reprinted and updated from *Idiot's Guides: Thyroid Disease.*

A WORLD OF IDEAS:
SEE ALL THERE IS TO KNOW

www.dk.com

Contents

Appendixes

Introduction

One out of 10 Americans is estimated to have thyroid disease. That's over 30 million people—more than the number of people who have diabetes. In contrast to other widespread illnesses, though, thyroid disease is a quiet epidemic. Many who suffer from it don't even realize they have it. That's because the thyroid regulates the energy level of your every cell, so when it malfunctions you can develop problems involving any part of your body, including your brain, heart, bones, skin, nails, and hair.

For example, if you have hypothyroidism—caused by your thyroid becoming underactive—you might find yourself gaining weight, feeling fatigued, growing confused, becoming depressed, developing rough skin, losing hair, feeling cold, getting acne, or experiencing any of dozens of other issues.

Alternatively, if you have hyperthyroidism—caused by your thyroid becoming overactive—you might start losing weight, feeling manic, growing anxious, getting panic attacks, having trouble sleeping, developing hand tremors, sweating excessively, developing eye problems, growing goiters in your neck, or experiencing your heart pound in your chest.

Thyroid disease symptoms can creep up on you so subtly and gradually that it takes months before you even recognize that you're ill. It often isn't until patients are treated and made healthy again that they realize all the ways their bodies had gone wrong. It's for this reason that some have called thyroid disease insidious.

Thyroid disease can be hard to diagnose, even by experienced doctors. Making things worse is a widespread lack of understanding about how to optimally interpret lab results, which medications are most effective, the enormous importance of diet, and common underlying conditions to look for beyond thyroid disease.

If you're experiencing thyroid disease symptoms and aren't sure what's causing them, this book is for you. It will guide you in identifying your symptoms, finding the right doctor, and getting the best testing and diagnosis possible.

Alternatively, if you already know that you have thyroid disease but are unsatisfied with your treatment, this book is very much for you as well. It will tell you how to analyze your lab results, choose the best medication, find the perfect dosage, and more.

Then again, if you have a friend or loved one with thyroid disease, this book will help you understand the pain it can cause and provide you with the information to help.

Whatever the reason you need thyroid information, this book will empower you to cut through the confusion, make informed choices, and embark on the path to full health.

How to Use This Book

The first four chapters of this book apply to everyone, and we recommend that you read them first. After that, you can skip around and focus on only the chapters that most interest you. There are plentiful cross-references to chapters throughout the book, and there's also a detailed index, so if you encounter a term or concept that's unfamiliar, you'll know which chapter to read to learn more about it.

This book's topics are organized into six parts:

Part 1, Getting to Know Your Thyroid, explains what your thyroid does and why it's so important to your health. It also describes symptoms that might indicate you have thyroid disease, controversies about thyroid diagnosis and treatment, and how to find a great doctor. It consists of Chapters 1-4.

Part 2, Hypothyroidism, details what to do if you're suffering from a shortage of thyroid hormones. It guides you step-by-step through identifying your symptoms, getting the precise tests you need (many doctors don't get this right), correctly analyzing your lab results (many doctors don't get this right either), choosing the best medication for your needs (most doctors don't get this right), and arriving at the perfect dosage to restore you to full health. It consists of Chapters 5-9.

Part 3, Hyperthyroidism, describes what to do if you're suffering from an excess of thyroid hormones. You'll discover how to recognize hyperthyroidism symptoms, get the right tests for it, analyze your lab results, and choose among the different treatments for it. It consists of Chapters 10-12.

Part 4, Other Thyroid Diseases, provides a step-by-step guide to dealing with thyroid cancer; managing thyroid-related problems such as adrenal gland disease and parathyroid disease; and treating ailments such as depression, anxiety, infertility, and severe PMS that can stem from a malfunctioning thyroid. It consists of Chapters 13-17.

Part 5, Healing Through Diet and Lifestyle, provides you with dietary suggestions that could end up slowing or even reversing your thyroid disease. It also offers a program for dramatically shedding inches off your waist. And it tells you how to avoid things that are harmful to your thyroid, including toxins and stress. It consists of Chapters 18-20.

Part 6, Underlying Conditions and Optimal Healing, covers diseases that might be afflicting you *in addition* to your thyroid disease, and offers guidelines for selecting top-notch thyroid doctors and other healthcare professionals. It consists of Chapters 21-22.

In addition, this book has two appendixes. Appendix A is a glossary providing brief definitions of medical terms, and Appendix B is a list of resources for finding thyroid healthcare providers near you, conducting research on thyroid disease, and learning more about thyroid medications.

Please Note

Please note that this book was written by two people, Dr. Alan Christianson (world-class thyroid physician and bestselling author) and Hy Bender (thyroid patient and top professional writer whose books have sold more than 1 million copies). The word "we" is used when advice is coming from both of us. When describing Alan's personal experiences as a doctor, though, "I" is used instead.

Please also note that this book contains stories about Alan's patients to bring the medical information to life. While the stories are all true, the names and select details have been changed to protect patient privacy.

Acknowledgments

Hy Bender: Hy gives his heartfelt thanks to all the wonderful healers, of every kind, who work tirelessly for light and life.

Dr. Alan Christianson: I would like to thank my family, my team at Integrative Health, and my close friends. Thanks also to my patients who encouraged me, as well as educating me every day by sharing their experiences and things they have learned. I greatly appreciate my parents who instilled a love of reading and of medicine in me at an early age and continue to guide me. I'd also like to thank another parent, David Frawley, who as an author has given me valuable direction and insight.

Thanks to my precious children, Celestina and Ryan. Thank you both so much for being patient when I took time for this book. I love you both, and I'm so excited to see you grow into such amazing people. Biggest thanks of all go out to my lovely wife Kirin who encouraged me to pursue my dreams and was also gracious in sharing my time with the book. My biggest wish is that all her dreams will come true. I love you, honey!

Trademarks

All terms mentioned in this book that are known to be or are suspected of being trademarks or service marks have been appropriately capitalized. Alpha Books and Penguin Random House LLC cannot attest to the accuracy of this information. Use of a term in this book should not be regarded as affecting the validity of any trademark or service mark.

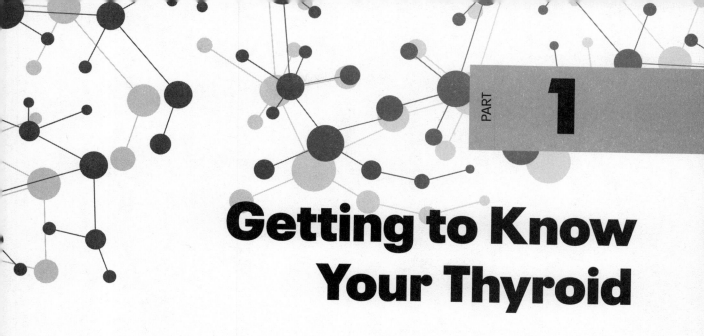

PART 1

Getting to Know Your Thyroid

In this part, Chapter 1 explains what your thyroid does, why it's vitally important to your health, and the ways it can go wrong.

Chapter 2 provides a checklist of thyroid disease symptoms so you can decide whether you have reason to suspect a thyroid problem.

Chapter 3 sheds light on various debates about thyroid diagnosis and treatment. It's important to have some understanding of the different views because many of the popular approaches to thyroid care aren't safe.

And Chapter 4 guides you in finding a great doctor and knowing what to expect from your office visits.

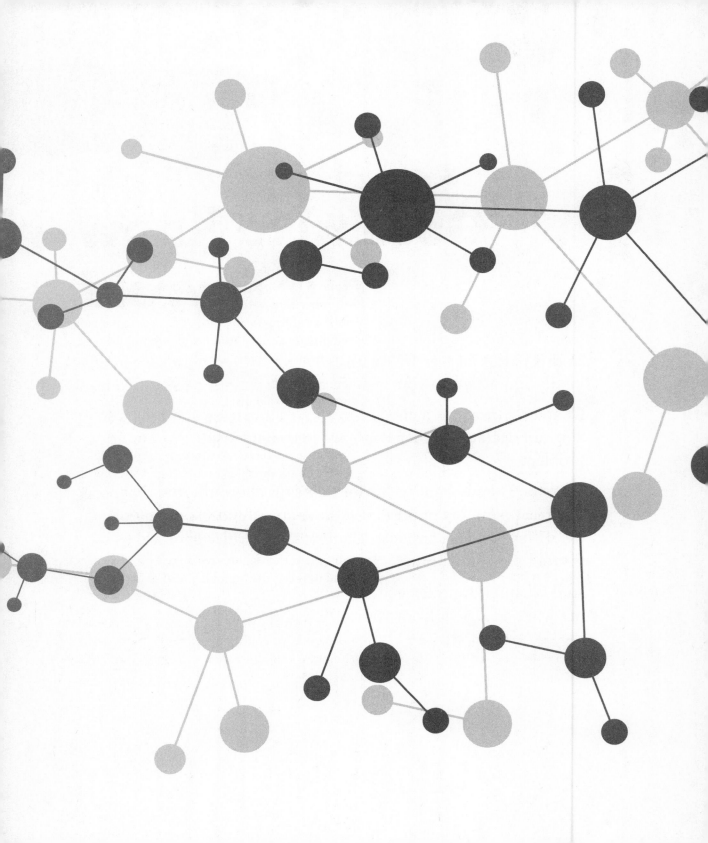

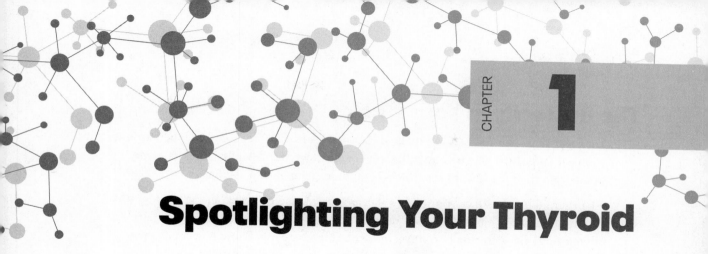

CHAPTER 1

Spotlighting Your Thyroid

Thyroid disease has become a quiet epidemic. The American Association of Clinical Endocrinologists (AACE) estimates 1 in 10 Americans have thyroid disease. That's over 30 million people—more than the number of Americans with diabetes. Women are over five times as likely to have thyroid disease as men. And the chances of having a thyroid disorder increase with time—17 percent if you're a woman, and 9 percent if you're a man, by the time you reach age 60.

The AACE also estimates that half of those with thyroid disease don't know it. That's because thyroid issues can be difficult to recognize, even by doctors. Many people suffer from thyroid problems for years before being accurately diagnosed. Further, even if you're receiving treatment for thyroid disease, there's a strong chance you're being underserved, because many doctors rely on too-broad lab ranges and outdated prescription habits, and fail to give sufficient weight to patient symptoms.

As alarming as the number of cases already is, the thyroid disease rate is expected to increase due to the thyroid's special issues with environmental toxins.

The good news is that almost all thyroid disease is thoroughly treatable. The challenge is to be fully informed, so you're empowered to recognize a problem and seek the right kind of help.

This chapter will take the mystery out of your thyroid. We'll explain what your thyroid is, what it does, and how it can go wrong. Whether you only suspect you have thyroid disease or are certain of it, you'll end up with the knowledge you need to start making informed choices and take appropriate next steps.

The Butterfly in Your Neck

Your *thyroid* is a butterfly-shaped gland that resides in your neck. It's wrapped around your windpipe, just above your collarbone and below your Adam's apple. Its name stems from the Greek word for "shield" (another metaphor for its shape).

The thyroid behaves like your body's thermostat, raising or lowering the amount of activity taking place based on your current needs. Your thyroid affects every part of your body by secreting hormones into your bloodstream. These hormones then charge up your cell's internal power batteries (more about this shortly).

Your thyroid consists of left and right "wings," called *lobes,* connected by a middle section called the *isthmus.* Your thyroid's two lobes do the same job, each performing half of the necessary labor. They also effectively back each other up. If anything goes wrong with one lobe, the other can take over the entire workload.

The thyroid's shape varies by gender. If you're a man, it's narrower and thicker; if you're a woman, it's longer and flatter. That's why the Adam's apple tends to be visible in men only. Women have an Adam's apple too—it's merely the cartilage between your thyroid and larynx—but the shape of the thyroid typically hides it from sight. (In fact, some ancient Greeks believed the purpose of the thyroid was to provide women with a pleasing neckline.)

Your thyroid isn't very large; it's roughly the width and thickness of four credit cards stacked on top of each other, and weighs 10–30 grams (0.35–1.06 ounces). Despite its relatively small size, though, your thyroid plays a critical role in your life.

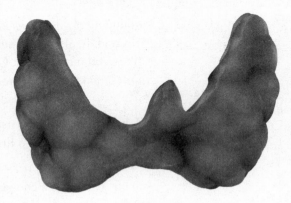

The thyroid gland
(Licensed from Shutterstock Images)

Your Energy Control Center

Your thyroid is one of the glands in your body's *endocrine system*. The thyroid has just one job, but it's of immense importance: it secretes a chemical, or *hormone*, directly into your bloodstream that regulates the energy level, growth, and reproduction of every cell of your body. That means your brain, heart, lungs, liver, skin, tissues, and all other body parts depend on your thyroid to stay "powered up" and active, and to remain healthy by generating new cells to replace old ones.

More specifically, each of your cells contains "power plants" called *mitochondria*. Simple cells contain just one, while more complex cells can contain several thousand mitochondria. Mitochondria take glucose (a fundamental sugar your body creates from the food you eat) and convert it into energy called *adenosine triphosphate*, or *ATP*. The cell then uses the ATP to fuel its activities, such as repairing your body, moving your body, firing thoughts in your brain, or reproducing.

How much or how little glucose the mitochondria convert into ATP is determined by the thyroid hormones circulating in your bloodstream. These hormones have a similar effect to your foot on a car's gas pedal, sending a message to either speed up or slow down. The mitochondria then function as little engines that convert your gasoline (glucose) into power (ATP) for driving your car (body).

The decisions about when to raise or lower cellular activity come from a portion of your brain called the *hypothalamus*. When your hypothalamus senses more energy is needed, it sends a chemical signal to an organ just above your sinuses that's about the size of a pea. This organ is called the *pituitary gland*.

Your pituitary gland then responds by producing *thyroid stimulating hormone*, or *TSH*, which is the chemical regulator of your thyroid. As its name indicates, TSH stimulates your thyroid, effectively telling it "We need more power. Get to work and make more hormones." Your thyroid then complies, making its hormones available to the mitochondria in each of your cells.

TSH is also an important diagnostic tool, because measuring its levels in your blood helps a doctor determine whether your thyroid is making too little of its hormones (TSH will be high) or too much (TSH will be low).

You can think about this energy management system as a company. The hypothalamus is the president, making "big picture" decisions about when to increase or decrease energy production. The pituitary gland is the vice president who relays those decisions. The thyroid is the company manager, sending out or holding back encouragement for energy production to each of the workers. And the mitochondria are the workers—and their activity has a huge effect because there are *trillions* of them.

The scenario is a little more complicated because various areas of your body can choose precisely when to make use of the thyroid hormones. It's as if your body is divided into different departments run by field-level managers, some of whom can decide whether the "speed up production" orders for the whole company are appropriate at that moment for that department. Overall, though, if your thyroid is churning out hormones, your cells will become more active.

Metabolism and Your Thyroid

The energy level set by your hypothalamus and enforced by your thyroid is called your *metabolism*. If you hear someone complaining that he's overweight because "I have a slow metabolism," he's saying that his thyroid is underactive. If that's truly the case, he should see a doctor. He might need thyroid medication (see Chapters 7–9), and/or he might be weight loss resistant (see Chapter 19). Then again, he might simply be eating too much and exercising too little (see Chapter 20).

As long as you're alive, your metabolism will never be set to zero. Even when you're doing nothing strenuous, your body needs to keep your heart beating, your lungs breathing, your brain processing information, and so on. A measure of this base level of activity is your *resting metabolic rate*, or *RMR*, which represents the minimum number of calories your body will use in 24 hours.

Your RMR is responsible for burning up 65–75 percent of your calories. While RMR varies based on weight, height, and age, as a rough rule of thumb RMR for an average woman is around 1,400 calories and for an average man is around 1,800 calories. And it's RMR that your thyroid is primarily designed to regulate.

Of course, you have some control over your body's energy management, too. When you choose to walk to work instead of drive, and to take the stairs instead of the elevator, you're sending messages to your brain to burn up more calories. Your hypothalamus will notice your demands for higher production, and set in motion the sequence of events that causes your cells to turn stored fat into glucose and then ATP.

Exercise and other physical activity typically burn up only 15–25 percent of your calories. (The other 10 percent is used up dealing with food.) However, intense exercise can raise your RMR for hours afterward, burning additional calories indirectly. Further, if you exercise regularly, you'll reduce fat and increase lean muscle, and *that* will raise your metabolism and RMR to a perpetual new high.

So while there's a lot of energy regulation going on inside your body that you don't directly control, you can opt for adjustments to your lifestyle to make this system accommodate your wants and needs...as long as your thyroid is healthy.

If your thyroid starts malfunctioning, however, it will typically throw off your RMR by a whopping 30–40 percent in either direction—roughly the equivalent of the number of calories you'd burn by running six miles a day. And a change in weight is only one of many problems you might experience, as we'll discuss later in this chapter.

The Iodine Connection

Your thyroid makes its hormones by combining two ingredients that you consume every day. The first is *tyrosine,* which is an amino acid that's found in many foods, such as bananas, avocados, white beans, wild rice, turkey, lean beef, fish, pumpkin seeds, sesame seeds, and almonds. You're likely to have plenty of tyrosine in your system.

The second is *iodine.* Your thyroid is unique in that it's the only gland that absorbs iodine; the rest of your body ignores this chemical. You require only a tiny amount of iodine daily: generally, 50–199 micrograms (mcg) (or 225–350 mcg if you're pregnant or breastfeeding). The iodine you consume quickly gets sucked into your thyroid.

Iodine availability in America has changed tremendously in the past few decades. While in the past people worried about not getting enough iodine, that's no longer an issue because iodine is so prevalent in our foods, seasonings, and medications. You're now far more likely to be struck by thyroid disease as a result of *too much* iodine.

Insufficient iodine is still an issue for many people in underdeveloped countries, but this problem affects fewer people every year. For example, as recently as 1990, 112 countries were severely iodine deficient. Now there are none.

Meanwhile, 30 countries are currently at risk for thyroid disease caused by iodine excess. The United States is among that 30.

To ensure you don't consume too much iodine—and to potentially start healing your thyroid—see Chapter 18.

The "T" Factor

Assuming you have enough tyrosine and iodine in your system, your thyroid makes its hormones in two basic steps. First, it induces a chemical process that converts tyrosine into *thyroglobulin,* which is a protein specifically designed to bind with iodine. Your thyroid then combines a thyroglobulin molecule with one to four iodine atoms. The number of atoms attached determines the type of thyroid hormone that results.

If your thyroid attaches four iodine atoms, the hormone *thyroxine* (also called *tetra-iodothyronine*) is produced. It's referred to as *T4* because it's made from a thyroglobulin molecule (T) combined with four iodine atoms (4). T4 comprises 85–90 percent of the hormones made by your thyroid.

T4 is a "storage" hormone. Instead of performing actions on your body, it's designed to circulate in your bloodstream, and be stored in your tissues, until thyroid hormones are needed by an area of your body.

When energy is called for, an enzyme named *deiodinase type 1* is used to strip off a single iodine atom from the outer ring of a T4 molecule. Deiodinase type 1 is stored in your liver, kidneys, brain, pituitary gland, muscles, skin, and tissues, which makes it rapidly available to every area of your body.

Converting T4 to a thyroid hormone with three iodine atoms results in *triiodothyronine,* or *T3.* And it's T3 that enters cells and "recharges" them by powering up their mitochondria in your cells.

It might seem wasteful to create T4 just so it can be transformed into T3. But T4 remains potent for about eight days in your bloodstream and tissues, while T3 retains its power for only around one day. So T4 gives each region of your body the flexibility of having a thyroid hormone constantly available and then "activating" it via conversion to T3 as needed.

In addition to T3 being created via T4 conversion, your thyroid makes T3 directly, although in much smaller quantities than T4. Your thyroid's T4-to-T3 production ratio is roughly 13:1. Put another way, around 8 percent of the hormones your thyroid produces are T3.

If your thyroid is underperforming, most doctors will prescribe a branded medication called *Synthroid,* or its generic version *levothyroxine,* which are synthetic versions of T4. This is based on the notion that because your body can convert T4 to T3, a pill with T4 is all you need. However, many thyroid experts argue that your thyroid must be producing both T4 and T3 for a good reason, and therefore, your medication should also be a mix of T4 and T3.

That's backed up by real-world experience. Roughly one out of three patients don't do well with T4 medication alone.

As a result, an increasing number of doctors are prescribing a combination of Synthroid and *Cytomel,* which is synthetic T3; or *desiccated thyroid* (also called *glandular thyroid, natural desiccated thyroid,* or *NDT),* which is a natural mix of T4 and T3 derived from the thyroid of pigs. To learn more and decide which option is best for you, see Chapters 3 and 8.

You should also know the enzyme deiodinase type 1 is made in part from the chemical *selenium.* If you happen to be low on selenium (which can be detected via blood tests), then your body won't be able to convert enough T4 to T3. The simplest solution is to eat a single Brazil nut daily. (Don't eat more than one a day regularly, as that could eventually result in a selenium overdose.)

T4 and T3 comprise around 96 percent of the hormones your thyroid produces, but they're not the whole story. Roughly 4 percent of thyroid hormones are *T2* and *T1.* As you've probably guessed by now, T2, or *do-iodothyronine,* is made with two iodine atoms. Until recently, most doctors considered T2 to be useless. However, some researchers didn't believe your thyroid would create something for no reason, so they took a closer look; their studies indicate T2 plays a role in metabolism and burning fat. It might also help with T4-to-T3 conversion.

Mono-iodothyronine, or *T1,* has no known purpose so far. But researchers are taking a look at it, too.

T2 and T1 are especially relevant when considering treatment. The only prescription medication that includes all four types of thyroid hormone is desiccated thyroid (sold under brand names such as *Nature-Throid* or *Armour Thyroid*). That means if your thyroid has entirely stopped working, or if your thyroid has been removed, desiccated thyroid is your only option for continuing to have a normal amount of T2 and T1 in your body. Your doctor might give you a hard time if you request desiccated thyroid, but the reasons she provides are likely to be historical ones that have been obsolete for decades (see Chapters 3 and 8).

One other thyroid hormone you might hear about is *reverse T3*. This is created when a batch of T4 is no longer needed (for example, after it's outlived its "expiration date" of potency, or when your bloodstream has too much T4). Just as your body creates T3 by stripping off an iodine atom from the outer ring of a T4 molecule, it creates reverse T3 by stripping off an iodine atom from the inner ring of a T4 molecule. The reverse T3 will then be flushed out of your body.

Some alternative medicine practitioners claim reverse T3 has special significance in diagnosing disease (see Chapter 3). However, to date the evidence doesn't support reverse T3 being notable as anything other than an efficient way for your body to dispose of T4.

When Thyroids Go Wrong

Your thyroid normally creates just the right amount of hormones for your body's current needs, keeping all your cells active and operating smoothly. If your thyroid becomes defective, though, you'll probably experience a bewildering set of disparate ailments because of the thyroid's pervasive impact on all parts of the body (see Chapter 2).

The three diseases that most frequently affect the thyroid are *hypothyroidism, hyperthyroidism,* and *thyroid cancer.*

Hypothyroidism

Hypothyroidism is by far the most common of thyroid diseases. If you're hypothyroid, your thyroid is underperforming—that is, failing to produce enough of its hormones. This shortage reduces your energy and impairs the function of cells throughout your body.

When your body doesn't have enough thyroid hormones, the mitochondria in your cells will reduce their conversion of glucose into ATP. The unused glucose will be stored in your body as fat, causing you to gain weight. You'll also start feeling increasingly tired as your energy supply winds down.

In addition, your body cutting down on the generation of new cells might cause your nails to grow dry and brittle, your skin to become rough and thin, and your hair to thin and fall out. At the same time, the lowered brain activity might make you confused, forgetful, and even dangerously depressed.

You can experience any of these symptoms, and/or dozens of others, because the "energy slowdown" caused by your underperforming thyroid will have different effects on different parts of your body.

Hypothyroidism is a complicated disease. With the help of this book, however, the chances are high that you'll be able to navigate the various difficulties and obtain treatment that resolves all your thyroid problems. To find out much more, see Chapters 5–9.

Hyperthyroidism

If you're *hyperthyroid,* your thyroid is overperforming—that is, making too much of its hormones. This accounts for roughly 15 percent of thyroid cases.

When your body has an overabundance of thyroid hormones, the mitochondria in your cells will turn glucose into ATP at a much faster pace than normal. Once the available glucose runs out, your body will start turning your fat cells into glucose to keep up with the mitochondria's demand for more fuel, causing you to lose weight. You might be happy about the latter. However, you'll also start feeling increasingly manic from the extra energy.

You might also feel exceptionally anxious, nervous, irritable, or "shaky," and experience tremors, severe anxiety, or panic attacks. In addition, your heart rate might dangerously increase to the point of pounding in your chest, which poses the risk of a heart attack.

Hyperthyroidism is a more dangerous disease than hypothyroidism, and it requires more complex treatment. However, in most cases it's thoroughly manageable. Treatment often requires time and patience until you either become healthy again or go in the other direction and become hypothyroid (which is a much easier disease to manage). For details, see Chapters 10 through 12.

Thyroid Cancer

The thyroid disease that causes the most terror is thyroid cancer. It's relatively rare, comprising less than 1 percent of thyroid disease cases. Still, that adds up to more than 50,000 Americans being struck by it every year.

Cancer has a reputation of being deadly and untreatable. Fortunately, that usually doesn't apply to thyroid cancer, which is about as treatable as cancer gets. The most common thyroid cancers, *papillary* and *follicular*, have a cure rate of 97 percent.

If you have thyroid cancer, your treatment will typically consist of surgically removing the thyroid and then giving you a dose of radioactive iodine. Because your thyroid is the only part of your body that absorbs it, the iodine will be ignored by the rest of your body and enter only whatever thyroid cells remain post-surgery—including all the cancer cells—at which point the radiation will obliterate them.

For a detailed description of diagnosing and dealing with thyroid cancer, see Chapter 13.

Other Thyroid-Related Problems

There are a number of other things that can go wrong in your body that either affect your thyroid or are affected by your thyroid.

For example, your thyroid does its job in partnership with your *adrenal glands,* which facilitate the conversion of T4 to T3, and allow T3 to enter cell membranes and access mitochondria. If your adrenals malfunction, lab tests will still show your thyroid to be working perfectly...because it is. But because your thyroid hormones are being blocked from doing their work, you'll nonetheless be hypothyroid. To learn more about this subtle problem, see Chapter 14.

Other ailments that are in some way connected to your thyroid include parathyroid disease, thyroiditis, thyroid eye disease, and MEN syndrome. For details, see Chapter 15.

Two special problem areas resulting from thyroid disease that often don't get enough attention are mental and emotional disorders, and women's issues such as PMS, fertility, perimenopause, and menopause. These are covered in Chapters 16 and 17.

Why Thyroids Go Wrong

Thyroid disease is as old as mankind. In ancient times, its primary cause was a lack of iodine. In our era we've done away with iodine shortages, but in our zeal to fix the problem created a brand new one: way too much iodine in our foods, medications, and supplements.

For example, a non-pregnant adult should stay typically within the range of 50–199 mcg of iodine per day, but it's easy to go way above that—especially if you eat a lot of dairy, baked goods, or seafood, use iodized salt, and/or take a standard multivitamin. Recent studies indicate these iodine overdoses might be the primary modern cause of thyroid disease. For much more about this, see Chapter 18.

Another issue is that your thyroid is extraordinarily effective at drawing in and storing iodine. If you aren't consuming excessive amounts of iodine, that's normally a good thing. However, dangerous substances such as mercury and perchlorate are chemically like iodine. Small amounts of such chemicals might find their way into your body via processed foods, pesticides on produce, poor quality water, and so on. If your thyroid mistakes them for iodine, it'll suck them up and store them, too.

Over time, the amount of unhealthy chemicals that accumulate in your thyroid can become so significant that they'll trigger your body's immune system. Your body will designate them as foreign invaders, and create antibodies to attack them so they can be flushed out of your system. Unfortunately, the antibodies might mistake your thyroid as an accomplice of the toxins (which, in a way, it is) and attack your thyroid cells.

This is called an *autoimmune* response, and it's believed to be responsible for many cases of both hypothyroidism and hyperthyroidism. Every year increasingly more chemicals are being pumped into both the environment and our food supply; and the older you get, the more toxins will accumulate in your thyroid.

That said, there are a number of things you can do to improve your chances of avoiding or mitigating thyroid disease. For approaches to healing that don't depend on medication, see Chapters 18 through 20.

Yet another problem in our modern age is low-level radiation, which is believed to be the primary cause of thyroid cancer (see Chapter 13). Complicating matters is that radiation is among the treatments for hyperthyroidism. For the pros and cons of pursuing this treatment, see Chapter 12.

Thyroid ailments might also stem from viral infections, allergies, food reactions, nutrient deficiencies, adrenal stressors, hormonal stressors, and more. You can learn about the different types of thyroid diseases and their causes in Chapters 5, 10, 13, and 15.

In addition, you can learn about diseases that sometimes lurk beneath a thyroid disorder in Chapter 21.

Now that you have a general understanding of your thyroid and how it can go wrong, you're ready to dig deeper. The next chapter describes the most common symptoms related to thyroid disease. It'll help you better understand what you're feeling, and also articulate those feelings in terms a physician will recognize if you choose to seek testing.

CHAPTER 2

Sorting Through Symptoms

Thyroid disease is often hard to identify because it can create any of dozens of wildly varying symptoms, ranging from weight change to insomnia to brittle nails to mood swings. Even superb doctors who don't happen to be experts in this area can fail to realize when a problem is being caused by an ailing thyroid.

The good news is we're here to help. In this chapter, we'll guide you through the most common symptoms of thyroid disease, complete with real-life stories about patients who had one or more of these issues and thoroughly overcame them with inexpensive thyroid medication.

Once you're done reading, you'll have a checklist of symptoms you can take to your doctor for testing, diagnosis, and possible treatment.

Hearing Your Thyroid's Messages

As explained in Chapter 1, your thyroid regulates the energy levels of your body by producing hormones that make your cells increase or decrease their activity. Because these hormones affect organs, tissues, and cells throughout your body, if your thyroid starts malfunctioning you might experience myriad problems stemming from your brain, your colon, your skin, your neck...the possibilities are overwhelming.

Some symptoms may be obvious, such as trouble swallowing or eye pain. Others can be so subtle—such as feeling irritable or becoming forgetful—that you're unlikely to immediately recognize them as the results of an illness.

Diagnosing thyroid disease is tricky for doctors. Different patients can have completely different symptoms, combinations of symptoms, and severity of symptoms, all stemming from an off-kilter thyroid.

There are millions of people who suffer from debilitating symptoms simply because neither they nor their doctors have recognized the root cause as a defective thyroid. It's a tragedy because thyroid disease is usually easy to treat...but not until it's been identified.

For example, I had a patient we'll call Margaret who'd been seeing me as her general practitioner for several years. During a routine check-up, I asked Margaret if she was sleeping well, and she casually replied, "I've been having insomnia." I noticed she looked a little too thin, so I checked her weight; it was down 14 pounds from the previous year. Margaret told me she wasn't dieting. "I just haven't been as hungry lately; no big deal," she said. I noticed she was sweating even though the room was cool, and her resting heart rate was a rapid 100 beats per minute. If I wasn't an expert on thyroid symptoms, I might have prescribed sleeping pills instead of putting the pieces together. Instead, I tested Margaret and, as I suspected, she was suffering from hyperthyroidism. Medication soon eliminated all the problems and restored Margaret to a happy life.

Too often we rationalize changes in our bodies, altering our perception of what's normal rather than acknowledging that there's something wrong.

This chapter will empower you to listen to your body when it's saying your thyroid isn't doing its job.

Thyroid Disease Symptoms Checklist

Because thyroid hormones affect every cell, in theory an ailing thyroid can result in any of hundreds of different symptoms. In general, though, certain symptoms are more likely to occur than others. These frequent clues to thyroid malfunction appear in the checklist that follows.

Take a few minutes to go over the list and check off any symptom that applies to you. If you aren't sure whether you have a symptom, find the description of it later in this chapter and use the additional information to make your decision.

Thyroid Disease Symptoms Checklist

- ○ Gaining weight for no apparent reason
- ○ Losing weight for no apparent reason
- ○ Frequent exhaustion
- ○ Sluggishness
- ○ Nervousness
- ○ Anxiety
- ○ Irritability
- ○ Feeling "shaky"
- ○ Slowed thinking
- ○ Memory problems
- ○ Depression
- ○ Lowered interest in sex
- ○ Excessive interest in sex
- ○ Menstrual problems
- ○ Infertility
- ○ Insomnia
- ○ Constipation

- ○ Unusually frequent bowel movements
- ○ Hair loss
- ○ Thinning or dry hair
- ○ Dry, brittle nails
- ○ Rough, itchy, and/or thinning skin
- ○ Acne
- ○ Puffy skin
- ○ Cold skin
- ○ Feeling unusually cold
- ○ Sweating too little or too much
- ○ Numbness or tingling in the hands and feet
- ○ Rapid heartbeat
- ○ Weak muscles
- ○ Painful and/or enlarged eyes
- ○ Hoarse voice
- ○ Enlarged neck

If you have six or more of these common symptoms, there's a strong chance your thyroid is ailing. Get your thyroid checked out—typically via blood tests for TSH, free T4, free T3, and antibodies—as soon as possible.

If you have two to five of these symptoms, that's still reason enough to get your thyroid tested. Either the results will be positive, putting you on the path to treatment, or negative, which will inform your doctor to explore other potential problem sources. (Before accepting a negative result, though, see Chapter 7.)

But even if you have only one of these symptoms, and your doctor isn't providing a satisfying explanation for its cause, you should seriously consider getting tested. That's doubly true if you're a woman who's 30–50 years old, because that's the gender and age range most often struck by hypothyroidism.

The checklist is by no means comprehensive; you can experience other symptoms. However, the odds are that along with the unlisted symptoms, you'll have at least a few of the ones on the checklist. If you're successfully treated for thyroid disease, you'll soon experience improvement regarding *all* your thyroid-related symptoms.

Virtually any symptom on the checklist can be caused by something beyond a faulty thyroid. Therefore, ask your doctor to give you a full physical, and to explore other potential causes *in addition* to the thyroid testing (see Chapters 14, 15, and 21). Even if your symptoms turn out to be entirely thyroid-related, that doesn't mean the search for causes should end. For example, if you have an autoimmune thyroid disease, it might have developed from toxins in your system. Eliminating such toxins (by changing your water supply, switching to organic food, etc.) could result in your eventually not needing thyroid medication...and lead to overall better health.

The rest of this chapter describes common thyroid-related symptoms in more depth, then concludes with some advice about testing.

Weight and Energy Symptoms

By far the most well-known symptoms of an ailing thyroid are weight gain and low energy (for hypothyroidism) or weight loss and excessive energy (for hyper-thyroidism). Both issues are related to your metabolism, which your thyroid can inadvertently set to operate too slowly or too quickly.

Gaining or Losing Weight

Your thyroid controls your resting metabolic rate (RMR), which is the minimum number of calories your body burns in 24 hours. To better understand this concept, think of your body as a car that never shuts off. When the car is moving, it burns up gasoline at a higher rate. But even when it's just idling, it's burning up a significant amount of fuel.

RMR for an average woman is in the neighborhood of 1,400 calories and about 1,800 calories for an average man. When an off-kilter thyroid changes your RMR by even just a third, it has an enormous impact on your body's calorie consumption.

If your thyroid suddenly starts underproducing hormones, your body's "idle" rate will go down, making you burn fewer calories per hour. This will cause you to gain weight...possibly a lot of weight. Even if you eat less and exercise more, it probably won't be enough to compensate for your lowered metabolism.

For example, Elizabeth was convinced her thyroid was off because she was struggling so hard with her weight. Noticing she was 5'9" and weighed 117 pounds, at first I thought she had a body image problem. Then she explained she thought her current weight was fine, but she was taking extreme measures to maintain it. Six days a week Elizabeth got up at 4 A.M., ran 10 miles, and then spent another 30–45 minutes at the gym before going to work. And her diet consisted primarily of fruits and vegetables, never exceeding 900 calories a day! That's all I needed to hear to be convinced testing was called for; and it turned out Elizabeth was indeed suffering from hypothyroidism. Once we got her on medication, she was able to maintain her weight eating 1,400–1,600 calories and no more than an hour of exercise daily.

Alternatively, if your thyroid suddenly starts overproducing hormones, your body's "idle" rate will go up, making you burn more calories per hour. This will cause you to lose weight. If you've been overweight, that'll be good news...temporarily. But over time, you'll become dangerously thin.

In either case, thyroid treatment will return your metabolism to normal.

Just because you gain weight doesn't mean you have a thyroid or metabolism problem. If you tend to eat a lot and don't exercise, a weight gain is to be expected. However, if you've maintained a steady weight and then suddenly start gaining with no change in your diet or exercise habits, then thyroid testing is called for.

Sluggishness or Exhaustion

If you're a workaholic getting by on six hours of sleep a day, it's no surprise you feel exhausted. But if you have a reasonable schedule and normal sleep habits, and for no apparent reason suddenly feel burned out daily, something's wrong.

See if any of the following statements ring a bell:

O You're pushing yourself just to get through the day.

O Activities you used to love are such a strain that you've stopped enjoying them.

O You've stopped exercising, socializing, and so on because you can't spare the energy.

O You crash in the afternoon, wanting to do nothing but sleep.

O When you get home from work, you feel so dead tired that all you can do is sleep.

If any item on this list resonates and there's no clear cause for the problem, seeing a doctor and getting tested for hypothyroidism is a good idea.

Mental Symptoms

It's obvious an ailing thyroid can cause physical problems. But what many people—including a fair number of doctors—don't realize is the profound effect the thyroid has on your mental health. Your brain is one of the organs most affected by thyroid hormones. When that supply is thrown off-balance, your thoughts and emotions may soon follow.

The next three sections cover thyroid-related mental issues that can wreak havoc on the quality of your life until they're identified and treated.

Depression and Anxiety

If you're experiencing depression, anxiety, or moodiness, you might find friends disregarding these feelings as being "just in your mind." You might even rationalize them yourself as being tied to outside circumstances, such as stress at work.

But if your mental difficulties are ongoing, and if you have other thyroid-related symptoms (fatigue, weight change, hair loss, etc.) along with them, you shouldn't hesitate to get tested. In fact, even if you have no other symptoms but you can't identify a cause for the problem, a thyroid test is worth doing.

For example, Brittany came to see me for anxiety. She said it was caused by her boss thinking nothing she did was good enough. Upon questioning her, though, I learned Brittany's performance evaluations were always positive, and she received a raise after every review. Clearly there was something else going on.

As we talked more, I learned Brittany was just as anxious about her relationships with friends, her personal safety, and various other areas of her life. Her anxiety had nothing to do with work or stress.

Brittany had undergone talk therapy with an experienced psychologist and had also tried anti-anxiety medication. None of it helped. The psychiatrist referred her to me to see if there was a possible physical cause. Brittany had no other symptoms, but because she'd reached a dead end, I saw no harm in testing her thyroid as part of a blood evaluation.

To my surprise, the lab tests were positive. It's unusual for thyroid disease to manifest with just one symptom; but as Brittany's case demonstrates, every now and then, it happens. And if I hadn't ordered those $50 tests (note, prices can vary), Brittany might have struggled with anxiety for years, wrecking her life.

Instead, over the course of four months I gently raised Brittany's dose of thyroid medication, and frequently checked her blood, until her levels normalized. Even with no therapy or other medication, the intrusive thoughts that disrupted her days virtually disappeared. On the rare occasion when Brittany felt anxious, she was able to make the discomfort go away simply by exercising.

Even worse than anxiety is depression, which is one of the most devastating diseases for one's quality of life. In the words of a patient: "The really odd part about this is there's nothing upsetting or unusual going on in my life. And yet I notice my mood has significantly shifted. I don't have any interest in things I did before, I have to force myself to do much of anything, and I'm not enjoying anything."

If you have depression along with other thyroid-related symptoms, get tested.

That said, there have been studies in which patients didn't test positive for thyroid disease but weren't responding to antidepressants. In these studies, T3 (in the form of Cytomel) was added to the mix of meds to see if it would help regardless. In most cases, it did. No data exists on whether doctors misinterpreted the lab tests (see Chapter 7) and the patients really had thyroid problems after all. At any rate, using T3 as a supplement to antidepressants is becoming increasingly common.

If your doctor is prescribing Cytomel as a supplement to other medication, make sure he's monitoring your thyroid blood levels via TSH, free T4, and free T3 tests. Otherwise you could end up with too much T3 in your system and start experiencing hyperthyroid symptoms.

Fogginess and/or Forgetfulness

Roughly 20 percent of the calories burned up during your resting metabolic state are used by your brain. If your thyroid hormones decrease, they'll set your brain to be less active and fire up less frequently. As a result, your thinking might slow down, leading you to feel foggy and unfocused.

You might also have trouble remembering even simple things like the names of people you know, where you put your keys, and what year it is.

There are other possible causes of these symptoms. But if they occur along with fatigue, depression, etc., have your thyroid checked.

Nervousness and/or Irritability

Nervousness, irritability, and shakiness are typically thought of as hyperthyroid symptoms—that is, the results of your body being too revved up. And, in fact, they are. But they can *also* be evidence of hypothyroidism—particularly if they're accompanied by anxiety.

Either way, if you have such symptoms and there's no other clear cause, get tested. The results will tell you precisely what's going on.

Having Trouble Sleeping

When your thyroid is malfunctioning, your mind might fill with disjointed thoughts. This can result in you having trouble falling asleep as your mind sorts through all the things you experienced that day and all the things you plan to do the next day. Alternatively, you might fall asleep normally but then wake up soon afterward because your brain is having trouble doing its normal nighttime job of processing information.

There's also some interplay between thyroid-related symptoms. For example, if you're suffering from fatigue, it could cause insomnia because you need to get "played out" to properly unwind and sleep at night. That can't happen if you're too tired to be active.

There are so many potential causes for a sleep disorder that this symptom by itself shouldn't make you think "thyroid." But it's notable when combined with other thyroid-related symptoms.

Sex and Fertility Symptoms

Thyroid hormones directly affect the gonads influencing ovary and testicle functioning. This can affect menstruation, fertility, and sexual feelings.

For example, if you're a woman with an underperforming thyroid, your ovaries might do a poor job of synthesizing estrogen and progesterone, causing your menstrual cycles to become irregular. In more severe cases, it might also cause dysfunctional heavy bleeding and make the ovarian lining inadequate for proper fertilization. The latter can cause infertility or lead to a miscarriage.

It's also quite common for hypothyroidism to affect sexual desire; when your thyroid becomes underactive, your libido often will, too. That's in part because of the connection between thyroid hormones and your sexual organs. In addition, when your metabolism slows down, you're likely to feel less energetic and enthusiastic about *everything*...including sex.

For example, my patient Sandra had a very active sex life with her husband for the first three years of marriage; her girlfriends referred to them as "the bunnies." But over the next two years, she lost interest. "It's gotten so bad," she told me, "that I've begun making secret marks on the calendar to remind me to initiate sex at least a few times a month. Otherwise it wouldn't even occur to me."

Sandra wanted to try testosterone therapy. I told her that we first needed to run tests to determine the root cause of the problem. To be thorough, I included a thyroid test; and to my surprise, even though Sandra had no other thyroid-related symptoms, she tested positive for advanced hypothyroidism. As mentioned previously, it's unusual for one thyroid symptom to appear in isolation—but it can happen.

After several months of treatment, I received a "thank you" card from a man I didn't know. It had nothing on it but an illustration of two rabbits lounging by a river. I checked the last name against my patient records...and realized it was from Sandra's husband.

Irregularity Symptoms

Your small intestine and colon form a very long tube lined by rings. Think about "the wave" crowds do at sports stadiums. That's sort of what happens in this tube; the first ring fires, followed by the next ring, and so on, coaxing undigested material through your body. This process is called *peristalsis,* and its intensity is regulated by thyroid hormones.

If you're hypothyroid, peristalsis will be sluggish. As a result, you might experience constipation. In addition, you might absorb more calories because food is lingering longer in your long intestine and colon, which means you'll gain weight even faster from eating the same amount of food as usual. Further, you risk being exposed to more toxins because bad chemicals that normally would be flushed out of your system quickly are instead sticking around.

Conversely, if you're hyperthyroid, peristalsis is sped up. This can lead to increased bowel movements and/or loose stools. In addition, the undigested food racing through your body doesn't allow enough time for calories to be absorbed adequately. This is a major reason for losing weight under hyperthyroidism.

Occasional constipation and excessive bowel movements aren't unusual. But if the problem is ongoing and no other cause is evident, your thyroid is worth considering as the culprit.

Hair, Skin, and Nail Symptoms

When you have hypothyroidism, your body is forced to make a choice. With limited resources to call upon, it focuses energy on vital functions, such as keeping you breathing, while diverting energy from nonessentials...which include keeping your hair thick and full, skin soft and supple, and nails strong and healthy.

These are structural parts of your body. Hypothyroidism won't make them break down any quicker, but it might greatly slow down the rebuilding process, leading to eventual degeneration. It's like a city neglecting its infrastructure. Everything will keep running, but over time it'll look increasingly awful.

Hair That's Thin or Falling Out

If your hair becomes dry or thin, that's notable for thyroid concerns only in combination with other thyroid-related symptoms.

If you're losing hair, though, the details become meaningful. When caused by hypothyroidism, hair loss won't be patchy or localized, but instead diffuse, even, and nonpatterned. And it will typically include the full length of the shafts and follicles, as opposed to hair merely breaking off.

Most importantly, the hair loss will happen at a substantially greater rate than what you were used to when your thyroid was normal.

The good news is your head has around 100,000 hairs. Even if you've started losing some due to hypothyroidism, it would take years before you became bald—and because you're reading this book, you'll be on thyroid medication long before that happens.

Even better news is that if you're treated within two years, the chances are all the hair you lost will grow back.

Rough, Itchy, and/or Thinning Skin

Your skin's cells have a very high rate of turnover; they're continually flaking off and being replaced. If your body's repair rate slows down, your skin will become rough, calloused, itchy, and/or thin—especially on your fingertips, hands, upper arms, and feet.

Acne

If your body's energy decreases, the reduced maintenance of your skin can cause fatty acids and other wastes to build up and clog your pores. This makes your skin more vulnerable to bacterial infection and might lead to various forms of acne, such as pimples, boils, whiteheads, and blackheads, even if you're long past the teen years usually associated with acne.

Puffy and/or Cold Skin

Hypothyroidism causes a fluid called mucin to build up right below the skin. This results in a puffy appearance.

Centuries ago, doctors didn't understand the role of the thyroid in disease, but they noticed when patients came in with swelling from mucin buildup so severe it could be spotted from across the room. In 1877, the condition was named *myxedema;* and to this day, you might see the term myxedema used interchangeably with hypothyroidism.

Because your metabolism slows down, there's less energy available to generate heat. This can make you feel cold and lower your skin's resistance to cold. For example, you might find yourself bringing a sweater along wherever you go because you expect to feel colder than anyone else in the room. The feeling of cold tends to be especially prominent in the feet and hands. You might also suddenly find yourself wearing heavy socks to bed, or wearing gloves when you've never needed to before.

Dry, Brittle Nails

There are numerous ways your nails might become dry, lined, brittle, and break easily. For example, if you switch to a restrictive diet, or if you develop digestive problems, your nails will be affected by a decrease in minerals such as zinc and by a decrease in protein. But if nothing's changed in your life, your nails going downhill may indicate a thyroid issue.

Other Symptoms

As mentioned previously, a malfunctioning thyroid can lead to scores of different problems. The next six sections cover some of the most common ones that don't fit neatly into any category.

Racing Heart

One of the most frequent symptoms of hyperthyroidism is a rapidly beating heart. In fact, if you start taking thyroid medication, a good doctor will ask you to pay attention to ongoing heart palpitations, because that's the most obvious sign your thyroid levels are getting too high and you need to scale back on the meds (in which case, you should contact your doctor about getting retested ASAP).

In the earliest stages of hyperthyroidism, you might not notice your heart beating more quickly during the day when you have lots of distractions, but you might become aware of it at night as you lie quietly in bed. As the disease progresses, your increased heartbeat will become more pronounced. At that point you shouldn't think twice about seeing a doctor.

If you're hyperthyroid, or suspect you are, avoid exercise until you've been fully treated. Normally exercise will take you from a resting heart rate of around 70 beats per second to 130 bps; but if your resting heart rate is abnormally rapid, exercise could raise it to a dangerously high level of 170–200 bps. And much worse, once your rate goes up that high, it might *stay* there even after you've finished your session. That's a risk not worth taking. Instead, skip working out until you're okay again.

Numb or Tingling Hands and Feet

Your thyroid regulates the rate at which your nerves conduct signals through your body.

If you're hypothyroid, your nerves might start conducting signals with less energy. This will slow down your reflexes, and might also cause sporadic numbness, especially in your hands and feet.

Conversely, if you're hyperthyroid, your nerves might relay signals with excessive energy. This can result in exaggerated reflexes, tremors, and/or sporadic tingling or pain, particularly in your hands and feet.

Weak Muscles

One of the paradoxes of thyroid disease is that certain conditions can be caused by both too little and too much thyroid hormones. And a prime example is weakened muscles.

If you're hypothyroid, your muscles are being told to reduce their activity. Because the body has a "use it or lose it" policy, this will sap their strength over time.

If you're hyperthyroid, your muscles are being told to get super-active; but at the same time, you aren't absorbing the nutrients you need to nourish them.

While the reasons are different, both conditions can produce the same symptom.

Irregular Sweating

Your sweat glands are regulated by thyroid hormones. As a result, if your thyroid is underactive, you might suddenly find yourself barely sweating under conditions in which you'd normally be pouring buckets. Conversely, if your thyroid is overactive, you might be sweating gallons for no apparent reason.

The areas of your body most affected are typically your underarms, hands, and back of your head. For example, if you normally go to the gym and sweat a ton under your arms, you could suddenly find your shirt is virtually dry after a workout. This makes it tougher for your body to expel heat and can make exercising uncomfortable. If this keeps happening and nothing else has changed, get tested.

Painful and/or Enlarged Eyes

Your eyes are vulnerable to a hyperthyroid state called *Graves' disease*. This can make you sensitive to light, feel a painful dryness or grittiness in your eyes, or experience double vision. Even worse, as the disease progresses it can make your eyes protrude, creating a "bug-eyed" look. But if you're diagnosed during the early stages, an experienced doctor can treat you to keep that from happening.

Enlarged Neck and/or Hoarse Voice

There are a couple of ways your thyroid can grow so large that it affects your neck and/or your voice. When your pituitary gland senses your thyroid hormone levels are low, it tells your thyroid to grow new cells to get production back on track. That's normally a good thing. But if your thyroid develops a problem and substantially underachieves, your pituitary gland will respond by telling your thyroid to grow a lot larger than is good for you. In this case, one or more growths from your thyroid (called *goiters*) may get so big that they create a noticeable bulge in your neck. Further, they might put pressure on your nearby larynx, or *voice box*, causing your voice to sound hoarser. They could even make you have trouble swallowing.

Alternatively, a thyroid can develop smaller bumps, called *nodules*. Sometimes these nodules do no harm; but sometimes they're indications of thyroid cancer (see Chapter 13). As nodules continue growing, they're eventually visible as small bulges in the neck.

If you see or feel anything growing in your neck, see a doctor without delay. It'll probably be very treatable; but the sooner you're diagnosed, the better.

When in Doubt, Get Tested

If you've read through this chapter, you might now be feeling as if every ailment under the sun is caused by a faulty thyroid. Naturally, that's not the case. For example, most people who have weight problems simply eat too much and exercise too little. And most people who are fatigued just aren't giving their bodies enough rest and loving care.

However, 10–20 percent of people with suspect symptoms probably *are* suffering from thyroid disease. As explained in Chapter 1, thyroid disease has become an epidemic. Because thyroid blood tests are quick, easy, and relatively inexpensive, if you have a reasonable suspicion that your thyroid is malfunctioning, it's wise to err on the side of caution and get yourself tested.

So don't hesitate to see a doctor. Beyond thyroid testing, a good physician will perform a thorough check to identify other problems that might be causing your symptoms instead of—or in addition to—any thyroid issues. For advice on finding and selecting a physician, see Chapters 4 and 22.

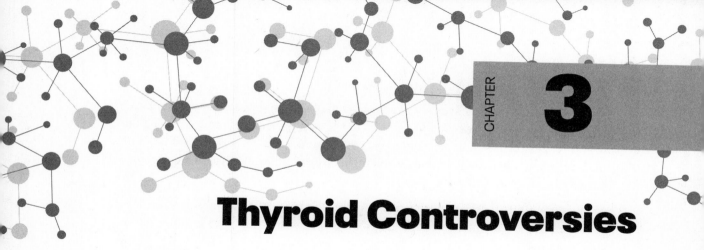

Thyroid Controversies

If you research thyroid disease online or skim through other thyroid books, you'll quickly be struck by the wildly different theories competing for your attention. Some will scream that mainstream doctors can't be trusted. Others will claim that alternative doctors are quacks. Some will declare that taking synthetic medication is insane. Others will tell you natural medication is unreliable. Further, each side makes an argument that, at first blush, sounds convincing.

These battling schools of thought can be terribly confusing even to experienced doctors, let alone a patient just starting to learn about the thyroid. This chapter will therefore gently guide you through the most common thyroid controversies you're likely to encounter as you explore potential physicians, talk to friends, and cruise the web.

Why the Thyroid Breeds Controversy

Few other medical problems inspire as much heated debate as thyroid disease. Part of the reason is the ubiquitous nature of the thyroid, which behaves like your body's thermostat, controlling how much or how little energy you receive. This affects dozens of functions throughout your system, ranging from how quickly you lose weight, to how much you want sex, to how happy you are. All this can make the thyroid appear to have mysterious and magical powers...and that mystical aura tends to attract eccentrics and quacks.

Further, the wide range and subtlety of thyroid problems can make them difficult to diagnose. There aren't many disease states whose very existence is debatable, and the frustration this creates for patients naturally leads to strong feelings and passionately expressed opinions.

There are also genuine issues involved. Many mainstream doctors have fallen into bad habits, such as focusing on blood tests to the exclusion of symptoms, relying on health ranges suggested by labs rather than by thyroid experts, and prescribing only high-priced synthetic medications when inexpensive traditional drugs often do a better job.

At the same time, there are alternative doctors who stray from sound scientific practices, or even common sense, championing approaches that pose serious risks to their patients.

Another reason for the heat is an evolution in the doctor-patient relationship. It used to be that your doctor told you what to do and you did it, no questions asked. Many modern patients aren't satisfied with such a one-sided arrangement; they want to actively participate in their diagnosis and treatment. And when it comes to the often-subtle symptoms of thyroid disease, that's appropriate.

What's unfortunate is that the discussion is so frequently framed as an "us against them" battle. There are extremely positive aspects to the strategies of both mainstream and alternative thyroid doctors, the views of both doctors and patient advocates, and so on. People tend to get in trouble when they cut themselves off from the perspectives of others and become tunnel-visioned.

The key to success for a good thyroid doctor is having a balanced approach. And that's the attitude you should take with each controversy: a healthy mix of openness and skepticism. As the saying goes, "Keep an open mind, but don't let your brain fall out."

Broda Barnes and Basal Temperature

One of the champions in the history of thyroid disease is Dr. Broda Barnes. Barnes was a prominent voice in correctly declaring hypothyroidism as a vastly underdiagnosed illness. He also pointed out that doctors fail their patients if they focus so much on lab test results that they neglect paying close attention to patient symptoms. And he was an advocate for desiccated thyroid medication at a time when this important option was in danger of being wiped out.

In addition, Barnes and his co-author, Lawrence Galton, wrote the seminal 1976 book, *Hypothyroidism: The Unsuspected Illness,* an exceptionally readable and compelling description of thyroid disease as Barnes understood it.

Barnes did fine work for his time; and his charismatic advocacy for a more organic approach to thyroid disease has won him followers who continue to use his methods. However, science has progressed since the days when Barnes practiced medicine. Certain techniques that he advocated 50 years ago simply aren't relevant in the 21st century.

Most prominently, Barnes advocated a diagnostic technique called the *basal temperature test*. This involved a patient placing a thermometer in his armpit for 10 minutes right after waking up. The reasoning was that a slowed metabolism results in a lower body temperature, and so a temperature of 97.8°F or below was evidence of hypothyroidism.

There are problems with this technique, though. Small variations in how a patient performs the test can create substantial differences in the result. There are other factors that can affect body temperature. And some temperatures Barnes considered evidence of a problem are now known to be normal for many patients.

Barnes developed the basal temperature test because the lab tests available in his time were woefully inadequate. Since then, however, medical science had made enormous progress. Labs can now process a small sample of your blood and provide remarkably precise and accurate information about how well or poorly your thyroid is performing.

So if you run across anyone who claims lab tests are useless and the only proper tool for diagnosing your thyroid's condition is the basal temperature test, that person is living in the past.

Along the same lines, if you learn a doctor you're considering bases her practice on the techniques of Barnes, seek a different doctor who has the same spirit of caring and attention to symptoms as Barnes did but who is also committed to using modern medical tools.

Wilson's Syndrome

In the late 1980s, E. Denis Wilson, a Florida doctor, declared he'd discovered a disease that was "the most common of all chronic ailments and probably takes a greater toll on society than any other medical condition." Rather immodestly, he termed it *Wilson's syndrome*. (You might also hear it called *Wilson's temperature syndrome* or *Wilson's thyroid syndrome*.) The symptoms described by Wilson echo those caused by thyroid disease—fatigue, hair loss, depression, and so on. However, Wilson claimed standard thyroid tests often don't pick up Wilson's syndrome because it's caused by an excess of reverse T3.

As explained in Chapter 1, your thyroid mostly produces T4, which can't be used directly but is a relatively long-lasting storage hormone. When your body is ready for increased energy, it removes a single iodine atom from the outer ring of a T4 molecule, converting the T4 to useable T3.

That's not the whole story, though. Your thyroid produces more T4 than you normally need. If your body doesn't end up using a T4 molecule by converting it to T3, it strips an iodine atom from the T4's inner ring to convert it to reverse T3. Reverse T3 is inactive and will simply be flushed out of your system.

Doctors don't normally test for reverse T3 because it's considered meaningless information, but Wilson based an entire theory of disease on reverse T3. Who's right? According to most reputable experts, not Wilson.

For example, back when Wilson first came out with his theory, I decided to check it out by having my lab run reverse T3 tests on more than 100 of my patients along with their standard tests. There was no evidence of elevated reverse T3 for any of my patients; the reverse T3 data proved to be random noise. In fairness, Wilson claims the problem can take place within cells, which wouldn't show up on blood tests. (In place of lab tests, Wilson relies on the Broda Barnes basal temperature test described in the previous section.) But if there's no hard evidence of a claim, how seriously can you take it?

Nonetheless, Wilson devised an elaborate treatment for his syndrome that involves escalating and decreasing doses of compounded time-released T3. For example, a dose might start at 5 mcg, work its way up to 100 mcg during a week, and then work its way back down again. The appeal of the process is that it's supposed to permanently cure all symptoms.

But aside from there being no reason to believe the treatment does any good, it's dangerous. In fact, one of Wilson's own patients died of heart failure after taking large amounts of thyroid hormones. In 1992, the Florida Board of Medicine suspended Wilson's license to practice. However, Wilson continues to write, lecture, and give seminars, and other doctors have taken up his ideas.

Guy Abraham's Iodine Project

According to such universally respected organizations as the U.S. National Institutes of Health (NIH), an adult should consume about 150 mcg of iodine per day (or 220/290 mcg if pregnant or breastfeeding), and shouldn't exceed 1,100 mcg (1.1 milligrams) of iodine daily.

Around three decades ago, however, Dr. Guy Abraham ran across some studies suggesting that megadoses of iodine could stop fibrocystic breast disease. These papers were recommending 5–20 milligrams a day—as much as 18 times what the NIH considers the maximum safe dosage. Abraham extrapolated from this that megadoses of iodine would be good for everyone...and especially patients with thyroid problems.

He blamed recommendations of 150 mcg per day on "iodophobia," a term he made up that refers to an irrational fear of iodine. According to Abraham, the right way to determine your appropriate iodine dosage is by swallowing a 50-milligram tablet of his own product Iodoral and then collecting your urine over the next 24 hours for testing. The rationale is that whatever iodine you don't pee out in a day is iodine your body must have needed.

After your first Iodoral experience, you're placed on a daily dose of it and periodically retested. Your iodine doses keep increasing until you're peeing out more than you're taking in. The problem with this process is that your body doesn't eliminate toxins with perfect efficiency (and at such high dosages, the iodine is indeed a toxin). It's a bit like giving you a high dose of mercury and then saying, "If you didn't pee it all out after a day, your body must be craving more mercury."

When your iodine intake abruptly increases, it can take months for your body to adjust and learn to expel the excess amounts in your urine. Meanwhile, overloading your thyroid with iodine can cause it to shut down, creating a state of hypothyroidism. Over time, it can also increase the risk of developing goiters, Graves' disease, Hashimoto's disease, or even thyroid cancer.

Nonetheless, a significant number of alternative medicine practitioners champion Abraham's theories.

Desiccated vs. Synthetic Medication

You might hear alternative medicine advocates proclaim that the only thyroid drug anyone should take is desiccated thyroid, such as Nature-Throid, WP Thyroid, or Armour Thyroid. Desiccated thyroid is prescription medication made from the cut-up and dried-out thyroid glands of pigs. It's the only medication available that contains all four thyroid hormones: T4 and T3 (in a 5:1 ratio), plus T2 and T1. Other names for desiccated thyroid include *natural thyroid, glandular thyroid, natural desiccated thyroid,* and *NDT.*

However, most mainstream doctors automatically prescribe Synthroid (or its generic version levothyroxine). Synthroid is created from chemicals in a lab and contains only T4. If you request desiccated thyroid instead, many of these doctors will refuse, or at least give you a very hard time before prescribing it.

This controversy results from a mix of historical and financial reasons. Synthroid first came on the market in 1955. Its manufacturer created an aggressive marketing campaign that touted it as new and modern, and portrayed desiccated thyroid as old-fashioned and inconsistent from batch to batch.

During this same period, there was a problem with a batch of desiccated thyroid that resulted in a patient being severely undertreated for hypothyroidism. This was reported in major medical journals, and it began turning mainstream doctors away from natural thyroid to the new synthetic wonder. The nail in the coffin for desiccated thyroid happened in 1970, when it was discovered most of the body's T3 comes from converted T4. (For further details, see Chapter 8.)

The problem was that the potency of desiccated thyroid medication at the time was determined by measuring iodine content. We now know this was a blunder because the amount of iodine in a pill can vary independently of its active hormones—most notably, its T4 and T3 content. As a result, these medications truly *were* inconsistent.

Since 1985, though, desiccated thyroid manufacturers have switched to measuring the exact amounts of T4 and T3 in their pills. They follow the guidelines of the United States Pharmacopeia (USP), which is a highly respected authority that sets public standards for medication. Synthetic drug companies follow these same USP guidelines.

Therefore, while their ingredients come from different sources—pigs for natural thyroid and chemicals for synthetic—both types of pills are formulated in labs following strict quality control procedures, and you can expect to consistently get the stated amounts of T4 and/or T3 in a pill regardless of its origins.

However, Synthroid generates much more revenue. It costs up to four times as much as desiccated thyroid, and its manufacturer holds a patent on it, while pig thyroid isn't something anyone can patent. Some have observed that the greater financial clout of Synthroid's manufacturer has been used to influence medical organizations to tout it above all other thyroid solutions. In fact, Synthroid is one of the most-prescribed drugs in the United States.

Which isn't to say Synthroid isn't an excellent medication. It is. And for a large percentage of patients, the T4 it provides does the job. Their bodies convert the T4 into T3, and the latter supplies all the energy they need. Plus there are some clear advantages to Synthroid. Because it's made from lab-based ingredients that are never likely to run out, it tends to stay readily available (barring manufacturing snafus), while there have been periodic shortages of the natural ingredients needed to make desiccated thyroid. Synthroid poses no problems for those who might be uncomfortable consuming pig-based products, such as Orthodox Jews and vegans.

Synthroid is available in the following microgram (mcg) dosages and pill color codes to meet any need for T4: 25 mcg (orange), 50 mcg (white), 75 mcg (violet), 88 mcg (olive), 100 mcg (yellow), 112 mcg (rose), 125 mcg (brown), 137 mcg (turquoise), 150 mcg (blue), 175 mcg (lilac), 200 mcg (pink), and 300 mcg (green). And in case you can't remember what a color represents, the pertinent dosage number is etched into each pill. Synthroid is available in the widest range of dosages of all thyroid drugs, which makes it easy to fine-tune how much medication you're taking daily.

However, a healthy thyroid produces not only T4, but also T3 (in a roughly 13:1 ratio). No one knows why, but it turns out that around 1 out of 3 people really do need direct T3 as well as the T3 converted from T4. (This is especially the case for patients whose symptoms include depression, as direct T3 often has an enormous beneficial effect on emotions.) The solution for these patients is to take medication that provides direct T3 in addition to T4.

If you're one of these patients and your doctor won't budge from prescribing synthetics, you can request that your Synthroid be supplemented with Cytomel, which is synthetic T3. Cytomel's strength starts to fade after about 10 hours, so it should ideally be taken twice a day (once in the morning and once in the late afternoon). For many patients, a Synthroid-Cytomel mix works.

It's also worth noting a healthy thyroid produces a certain amount of T2, which research indicates plays a significant role in metabolism and weight loss. Studies show that, all things being equal, patients taking synthetic medication have less than half the T2 of patients on desiccated thyroid. In other words, even if your body is converting T4 to T3 efficiently, it's probably not also converting enough of that T3 to T2. The only medication on the market that provides T2 is desiccated thyroid.

(Desiccated thyroid also contains T1, which doesn't appear to do anything useful, but it might serve some function no one's discovered yet.)

Therefore, if you haven't started taking thyroid medication yet—or you have, but aren't satisfied with the results of your T4-only pill—and you have a good relationship with your doctor, you shouldn't hesitate to choose desiccated thyroid. It's just as reliable as Synthroid, costs substantially less, and is the only medication that provides all four thyroid hormones.

One other way to go is taking a combination of Synthroid (or its generic version levothyroxine) and desiccated thyroid. This allows you to adjust your T4:T3 ratio closer to the 13:1 ratio a human thyroid provides (see Chapter 9). There's no problem with mixing these medications; it's analogous to getting your daily vitamin C from eating two oranges, or by eating one orange and taking a vitamin pill.

There's no absolute right or wrong answer to this controversy; people have different body chemistries and different needs.

That said, if you choose to take desiccated thyroid but have trouble persuading your current doctor to prescribe it for you, you can use the "Finding Thyroid Healthcare Providers Near You" section of Appendix B to discover local doctors who will.

Brand Name vs. Generic Medication

If you're using desiccated thyroid, you don't have to make brand name versus generic decisions. The brand names are already so inexpensive that no generics even exist.

If you're considering synthetic medication, though, such brands as Synthroid (T4) and Cytomel (T3) can be three times as expensive as their generic versions of levothyroxine (T4) and liothyronine (T3) . Many patients swear they do significantly better on a brand name medication. Sometimes this is just their imagination. A perfect example is those who passionately declare WP Thyroid superior to

Nature-Throid, or vice versa. The truth is that both medications come from the same manufacturer, RLC Labs, and are identical.

They didn't start out that way. WP Thyroid (on the market since 1934) originally had filler ingredients that caused some patients allergic reactions, so in the 1960s RLC came out with a hypoallergenic version named Nature-Throid. Eventually, RLC decided to do away with WP Thyroid's allergic filler and use the exact same active and inactive ingredients for both medications.

That doesn't mean patients who champion WP Thyroid over Nature-Throid are lying, though; the strength of their belief that one brand is superior to the other gives them a better experience with that brand.

Then again, sometimes patients really *are* better off with a brand.

The active ingredients in thyroid pills are minute—a fraction of the size of a grain of salt. Most of a thyroid pill therefore consists of inactive ingredients that serve as filler. While the active ingredients are the same in both brand name and generic versions, the fillers will vary...and will have different effects on how well or poorly the active ingredients are absorbed by your body.

Further, the same pill might be absorbed efficiently by you but be poorly absorbed by someone else, because each person's body chemistry is unique. (It's for similar reasons you're told to take your thyroid medication on an empty stomach and wait 30–60 minutes before eating. Anything you consume might unexpectedly bond with the medication and prevent it from being absorbed.)

Therefore, the main advantage of buying a brand name is that you know what to expect. Unless the manufacturer changes the formulation, your pills will contain the same inactive ingredients every month; so even if you aren't absorbing a pill with maximum efficiency, it won't matter because your doctor will simply raise your dosage until you're always getting the amount of medication you need.

If you buy generic, though, there's a chance your pharmacy will obtain your pills from a different source in any given month. That means you could absorb the active ingredients efficiently one month and poorly the next—effectively changing your dosage without your knowledge.

That said, if you give generics a chance, you might find your body isn't very sensitive to changes to inactive ingredients. Or you might discover that your local pharmacy uses the same generic source month after month, providing you with the same consistency as the brand-name version.

If you want to save $10–$30 a month, you're not at great risk by trying generics. But if you go this route, pay extra attention to how you're feeling, and don't hesitate to see your doctor for another blood test if you believe your symptoms might be returning.

Also be aware that occasional manufacturing snafus will cause a thyroid medication to be recalled or to be temporarily taken off the market. This happens regardless of whether a thyroid medication is natural or synthetic, or a brand name or generic. The issue often isn't the source of the hormones, but the extreme precision required to make any thyroid pill that meets or exceeds USP specifications.

Standard vs. Compounded Medication

Some doctors aren't satisfied with thyroid drugs as they come from their manufacturers, and instead have a local compounding pharmacy create a version customized to their specifications—typically, by putting the medication into a time-released form, so it's more effective throughout the day. The reasoning is that while T4 is long-lasting, T3 loses its optimal strength relatively quickly.

However, if you're on desiccated thyroid medication such as Nature-Throid, the T3 will typically last most of the day; and because you're taking it daily, that's good enough.

Alternatively, if you're on Cytomel, its T3 will stop being optimal in your system after about 10 hours. If you find yourself fading out in the middle of the day, though, you can address this by taking half of your Cytomel dosage in the morning and the other half in the late afternoon.

It's true that a compounded, time-released thyroid medication provides extra convenience. But the risk isn't worth it. For example, a patient of mine we'll call Stella was doing well on standard thyroid medication. She then became convinced by another doctor that he had better ideas, and she switched to him. A few months later I received a call from Stella over the weekend, and it quickly become obvious to me that she was suffering from severe hyperthyroid symptoms. I urged Stella to go straight to the ER. When she was admitted, the hospital found her T3 levels were hundreds of times above normal. Stella ended up spending several months in a coma and on a respirator, and for a while it didn't seem as if she'd survive.

What happened is that the other doctor prescribed Stella a compounded mixture of T3 in a time-released form. The dosage was supposed to be 7.5 micrograms. However, the pharmacist made a mistake and instead created a dosage of 7.5 *milligrams,* or *one thousand times* as much. You might wonder how such a blunder could happen, but both a milligram and a microgram are smaller than a grain of salt. When dealing with such minute quantities, errors can and do occur. In fact, Stella was lucky. Other patients have died from similar accidents with compounded thyroid medication.

It's possible you'll end up taking thyroid medication every day for the rest of your life. If so, using compounded medication means you'd be allowing 365 chances a year for a pharmacist to make a serious mistake. Considering that the convenience factor is small and there's a risk of a fatal outcome, we recommend staying away from compounded thyroid medication.

To be clear, there's nothing wrong with compounding pharmacies. Most other medications aren't in quantities as minute as thyroid hormones and so don't involve the same degree of danger. Also, not every doctor who prescribes compounded thyroid is a quack. Some just haven't thought through the ramifications. Still, if you're considering a doctor who follows this practice, take an extra careful look at what else that doctor is doing.

Thyroid Medication Substitutes

As you cruise the web or visit health food stores, you might find people touting over-the-counter substitutes for thyroid medication. These products are desiccated thyroid derived from pigs or cows, but with the fat extracted. Hormones are concentrated in the fatty acid of the glands, so removing the fat eliminates most of these products' active hormones. Obviously, that makes these products much less effective. If the bulk of the active hormones could remain, however, the USDA would consider these products drugs—which means you wouldn't be able to buy them over the counter.

The ingredient lists of these substitutes imply that if you consumed about a dozen tablets, you'd be getting the rough equivalent of 1 grain (65 mg) of Nature-Throid. Even if that's true, it's a pretty inelegant way of taking thyroid medication. More importantly, these products aren't regulated remotely close to the standard of thyroid medication, so the dosing is likely to be inconsistent.

Also, because cow thyroid is sometimes used, and that thyroid is exposed to the brain during the slaughtering process, there's a small but real risk of contracting bovine spongiform encephalopathy (commonly known as mad cow disease). In other words, desiccated thyroid is a great product...but only via prescription.

There are also a number of over-the-counter products that claim to enhance thyroid function by focusing on iodine. While iodine truly is a key component for thyroid hormone production, most people are already consuming *too much* of it; plus there's reason to suspect excess iodine plays a role in causing thyroid disease (see Chapter 18).

Many over-the-counter supplements are wonderful. But steer clear of those that try to provide you with unregulated thyroid hormones or superfluous iodine. Instead, work with a doctor who can prescribe thyroid medication produced under strict quality control procedures; and who can also regularly check your blood's thyroid levels, provide an objective view of your symptoms, and keep an eye out for any additional issues.

If you don't already have a doctor who can test, diagnosis, and treat whatever ails you, the next chapter will guide you in finding one.

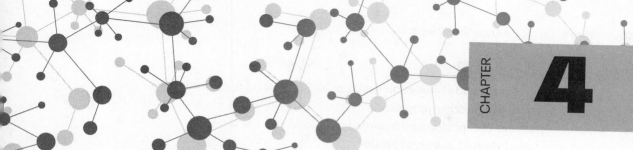

CHAPTER 4

Choosing the Right Doctor

Most major illnesses tend to be handled consistently and well throughout the medical community. In these cases, you don't have to worry about which doctor to choose, because you're likely to receive a comparable level of care from any good doctor.

Unfortunately, that's not the situation when it comes to thyroid disorders, which can make even skilled and caring physicians fumble. Thyroid diagnosis and treatment are moving targets, and what doctors are taught in medical school typically doesn't match up with the best practices of thyroid experts. Further, because the thyroid can cause any of dozens of seemingly unrelated symptoms, it's easy for doctors who aren't highly experienced with the thyroid to misinterpret the cause of a patient's problems...or even dismiss those problems as being nothing more than the patient's imagination.

As a result, if you don't take an active role in ensuring you have the right thyroid practitioner for your needs, you might be playing Russian roulette with your health. This chapter guides you in understanding your options, what questions you should ask, and what behavior from your doctor indicates you're receiving optimal care.

Initial Considerations

If you have reason to suspect a thyroid disorder—for example, if you have one or more of the symptoms described in Chapter 2—you should get your blood checked to determine your thyroid's status. Specifically, your doctor should take blood samples and instruct a lab to test them for at least three things: TSH, free T4, and free T3. The meaning of these tests is detailed in Chapter 7 (for hypothyroidism) and Chapter 11 (for hyperthyroidism). For now, what you need to know is that some less-savvy doctors will order only a TSH test; but the TSH, free T4, and free T3 tests are *all* required to provide adequate information about your thyroid's condition.

In addition, a sharp doctor will usually tell the lab to perform a one-time check for thyroid antibodies. These are indicators of such conditions as Hashimoto's and Graves', which are the most frequent causes of thyroid disease.

Virtually any doctor can take your blood and send it to a lab, so you might find it easiest to begin with a general practitioner you already know and trust. Then again, if you want to be in the hands of a specialist from the start, you should seek out an *endocrinologist*.

An endocrinologist is a doctor who specializes in disorders of the glands of the endocrine system and their hormones. These glands include the thyroid, parathyroids, pancreas, ovaries, testes, adrenal, pineal, pituitary, and hypothalamus.

For example, the most common illness treated by endocrinologists is diabetes, which is typically caused by the pancreas not producing enough insulin. And the next most common illness is hypothyroidism, which is typically caused by the thyroid not producing enough thyroid hormones.

Regardless of the type of doctor you see, your physician should carefully question you about your symptoms, conduct a thorough physical examination of your thyroid, and perform at least a brief overall physical exam.

If your doctor then wants to run tests beyond the thyroid blood tests, that's fine. In fact, it's often the responsible thing to do, because your symptoms might be stemming from something that has nothing do with your thyroid. Alternatively, your symptoms could be caused by multiple problems that include but aren't exclusive to your thyroid (see Chapters 14 and 21).

Here are some early warning signs that should make you seriously consider switching to a different doctor:

○ You're told to ignore a symptom— "It's just in your head" or "Reduce your stress and it'll go away." It's possible that's true, but there's no way to be sure until you're tested.

○ You're told the only tests you need don't involve your thyroid. It's fine to test for other things, but this should be done *in addition* to checking your thyroid hormone levels. Thyroid tests are only around $50 each and are covered by virtually all insurance plans, so there's no good reason to not perform them.

O You're told that the only thyroid test needed is the TSH test. That's the sign of a doctor out of touch with modern thyroid diagnosis methods. You can either insist on having free T4, free T3, and thyroid antibody tests included until the doctor complies, or you can say "thanks but no thanks" and seek a physician with more up-to-date knowledge.

If your doctor doesn't do any of these things, then you're probably in good hands. Before you end your visit, however, ask if you can be emailed, faxed, or mailed the thyroid test results after they come in from the lab.

Tip: If your doctor's office sends results by only fax and you don't have a fax machine, you can subscribe to a service that converts a fax into a PDF attachment that's emailed to you. This allows you to conveniently store all your medical test results permanently on your computer. An excellent affordable service is MyFax. com, which is free for a 30-day trial period and then $10 a month.

Be tactful when making your lab results request, indicating that you know a little about what the numbers mean (which you will after reading Chapter 7 or Chapter 11).

If your practitioner seems a bit put off by the request, that's not unusual, as doctors are accustomed to being fully in charge. But dealing with thyroid issues is a genuine collaboration between doctor and patient, and the best thyroid practitioners understand that. Be polite and diplomatic, and there shouldn't be a problem.

If your doctor flat-out refuses, that's another warning sign. In this case, ask if you can alternatively receive a photocopy of the results when you come in for your next visit. If you receive another no, then cancel the test and seek another doctor. You own your medical information and are legally entitled to it upon request. A doctor who denies your right to your lab data is also likely to deny your right to participate in your treatment.

Please also be aware that if your doctor detects one or more noticeable growths on your thyroid—that is, large enough to be seen and/or felt in your neck—then regardless of the results of the blood tests, you must have these checked out, too. Your doctor can begin by prescribing an ultrasound exam, which is quick, inexpensive, and poses no health risks. If the results don't clearly show the growths to be benign, there's a small possibility of thyroid cancer. For safety's sake, you should follow up by seeing an experienced ear, nose, and throat surgeon (see Chapter 13).

Your Second Visit

If you asked for your thyroid test results to be sent to you, then (typically) within a week you'll receive a page with some numbers on it from your doctor's office.

To understand these results, read Chapter 7 (if you think you're hypothyroid) or Chapter 11 (if you suspect hyperthyroidism). It will explain:

O What all the test numbers mean

O The TSH range used by the lab, which we'll call the *broad range*

O The TSH range that savvy thyroid experts use, which we'll call the *narrow range*

If your TSH falls within the narrow range, then you probably don't have a thyroid problem. If your TSH falls outside of the broad range, then you probably do; and your doctor won't need any convincing to treat you with thyroid medication.

If your TSH falls between the narrow and broad range, however, you're in a gray area that will make your diagnosis complicated. In this case, your doctor should pay extra careful attention to your free T3, free T4, and thyroid antibodies results. She should probably also order an ultrasound scan to see what's physically happening with your thyroid.

Most importantly, she should look beyond the numbers to your symptoms. If your symptoms persist and no other clear cause is identified for them, then you should be treated for thyroid disease regardless of the lab numbers. There's no significant downside to treatment; and if you really do have a thyroid problem, then within 2–6 weeks you should start feeling better.

Having this knowledge makes you an informed patient, and empowers you to both understand and evaluate your doctor's choices. When you see your doctor again, listen carefully as she discusses your thyroid test results and notice whether what she's telling you matches up with your own understanding. If you're confused, don't be shy about asking questions. (Sometimes doctors make shocking mistakes—for example, interpreting a high TSH to mean you have high thyroid levels when it means the opposite.)

If your TSH happens to fall into the gray area between the narrow and broad ranges, also pay attention to whether your doctor dismisses the possibility that you have thyroid disease. If this occurs, mention that the TSH range recommended by the American Association of Clinical Endocrinologists (AACE) indicates you're at risk, and that you don't believe your symptoms are just your imagination. If your doctor dismisses this as well, then you need to find another doctor.

Alternatively, if your physician demonstrates she has a balanced view by taking both the lab numbers and your symptoms into consideration, and by not treating the lab's recommended ranges as gospel, then the chances are she's the right doctor for you.

Considering Treatment Options

If your doctor decides that you need thyroid treatment, then your next discussion should be about medication. If you're seeing a mainstream doctor, he'll probably prescribe Synthroid (or the generic version levothyroxine), which is lab-created T4. Many patients will do fine on Synthroid. However, roughly 1 out of 3 will not.

The problem is that a healthy thyroid produces both T4 and T3 (in a roughly 13:1 ratio), but Synthroid is exclusively T4. Many patients will therefore do better on a mix of Synthroid and Cytomel (which is lab-created T3), or on desiccated thyroid such as Nature-Throid (natural thyroid taken from pigs, providing a mix of T4, T3, T2, and T1). More information about these medications can be found in Chapters 3 and 8.

Therefore, it's entirely appropriate to ask your doctor to prescribe desiccated thyroid instead of Synthroid; or if you prefer going with synthetics, to add Cytomel to the Synthroid. If he scoffs at your request and replies that Synthroid is always the best choice, then he's not giving you accurate advice, but don't be too hard on him; he's merely echoing what he was taught in medical school. If you find he's a good doctor in all other ways, then you might want to give him a chance and see if you do well on the Synthroid.

One exception is if your thyroid has entirely stopped functioning or has been removed, which means you're relying exclusively on your medication to provide the thyroid hormones your body requires. In this case you're better off with desiccated thyroid medication such as Nature-Throid, because desiccated thyroid is the only option that will provide you with the full range of thyroid hormones—that is, T4, T3, T2, and T1. If your doctor won't agree to your preference for medication, then you can start on Synthroid (which will do no harm), but you should also begin looking around for a different practitioner who'll accommodate you.

If you need help locating an appropriate doctor in your area, use the website resources listed in Appendix B. These range from online patient recommendations of thyroid physicians to free searchable databases containing information on hundreds of thousands of doctors.

For example, you can find doctors who regularly prescribe desiccated thyroid through the American Association of Naturopathic Physicians. (A naturopathic doctor has studied most of the same techniques as conventional doctors, but also uses alternative treatments such as herbal medicine and nutrition.) The Naturopathic.org website features a "Find an ND" button that allows you to search for doctors by location, telemedicine availability, and/or specialty (choose the "Endocrinology" option).

You can also get recommendations for alternative doctors through compounding pharmacies in your area, as these pharmacies typically stock desiccated thyroid. This is a bit tricky, however, because you don't want a doctor who prescribes compounded thyroid medication (see Chapter 3).

Follow-Up Visits

Once you've begun treatment, your doctor should see you every 1–2 months until your condition appears to be stable.

First, your doctor should keep taking your blood to check your TSH, free T4, and free T3 levels. The initial dosage you were given was essentially your doctor's best guess. These subsequent visits will allow your doctor to fine-tune your dosage based on your test results. This is a trial-and-error process, so it might take months of mild adjustments until your doctor finds the dosage that's perfect for you (see Chapter 9).

In addition, at each visit your doctor should perform a quick physical exam and question you about how you're feeling. If your symptoms are getting increasingly less severe, or have entirely disappeared, then the medication is working. But if that's not happening, you shouldn't hesitate to say so. What really matters aren't lab numbers but whether your symptoms are being successfully treated. The latter is the most important indicator of your health and what your doctor should focus on.

If your doctor refuses to make treatment adjustments even though your symptoms show no signs of improvement, then have a frank discussion about your concerns. If you aren't satisfied by your doctor's answers, seek a more diligent practitioner.

Beware Extremists

A thyroid doctor who takes a hardline approach in any direction is likely to be problematic. This chapter has already warned against mainstream doctors who believe Synthroid is the only appropriate medication for all thyroid patients. But you should also be wary of alternative doctors who proclaim that Nature-Throid is the only acceptable treatment. For example, if you require a finely tuned combination of T4 and T3, then a mix of Synthroid and Nature-Throid, or Synthroid and Cytomel, might prove to be ideal.

Here are some other approaches from alternative thyroid doctors that should set off alarm bells:

- **No blood tests.** If a doctor claims blood tests are unreliable, he's living in the 1950s. Thyroid tests really were lacking decades ago, but modern tests are accurate and invaluable tools.

- **Prescribing iodine.** There's no solid evidence that extra iodine does any good; and there's reason to believe it's dangerous, raising the risk of developing Graves' disease, Hashimoto's disease, or thyroid cancer (see Chapter 13).

- **Prescribing way too little thyroid medication.** Some doctors outrageously underprescribe; for example, by telling patients to take their thyroid medication once a week instead of daily. This not only fails to cure symptoms, it stresses the endocrine system more than if no medication was provided.

- **Prescribing way too much thyroid medication.** Typically, you shouldn't take much more than 1 mcg of T4 per pound of your body weight. Some alternative doctors instruct their patients to take four, five, or even six times as much thyroid medication as necessary. Over time this puts patients into a hyperthyroid state, which can lead to heart failure, accelerated osteoporosis, and other deadly disorders.

○ **Treating reverse T3.** Some alternative doctors subscribe to a theory called Wilson's syndrome that focuses on a byproduct of T4 called reverse T3, and which they treat with a T3 megadose (see Chapter 3). There's no solid evidence to support these ideas, and the treatment is so dangerous that it's caused deaths. Stay away.

○ **Prescribing compounded medication.** There's usually nothing wrong with compounded drugs—that is, medication prepared by a local pharmacy to a doctor's specifications. However, it's dangerous when it comes to thyroid medication, because the active ingredients in thyroid pills are so minute that even a small mistake by a pharmacist can result in an enormous overdose. Patients have died from such errors.

Additional details about these practices appear in Chapter 3. The bottom line is you should steer clear of doctors with these wrong-headed approaches, which have little connection to medical science and can put your health at serious risk.

Instead, look for a doctor who is open-minded and has a balanced approach. If you're exploring mainstream doctors, look for one who instead of focusing solely on lab results also pays careful attention to your symptoms and to how you're feeling. And if you're considering alternative doctors, look for one who makes full use of modern medical tools such as thyroid blood tests and doesn't advocate wacky theories.

When it comes to thyroid care, a nuanced, middle-ground approach produces the best results.

For further information on choosing the right doctor, and to also consider signing on with a team of healthcare providers, see Chapter 22.

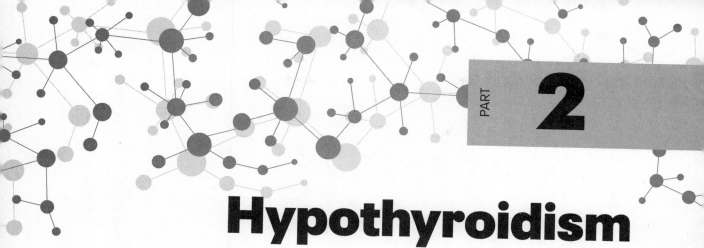

PART 2

Hypothyroidism

In this part we focus on hypothyroidism, which is typically caused by an underactive thyroid and comprises the vast majority of thyroid disease cases.

Chapters 5 and 6 explore potential causes for the disease, describe its symptoms, and tell patient stories that bring the medical information we've covered to vibrant life.

Chapter 7 explains the thyroid blood tests you need (many doctors order incomplete testing), and details how to obtain and analyze your lab results (most doctors interpret test results using lab-supplied ranges but instead should be using optimal ranges).

Chapter 8 tells you about your medication options, and why what most doctors automatically prescribe probably isn't the best choice for you.

And Chapter 9 guides you through the process of determining your perfect dosage for optimal health.

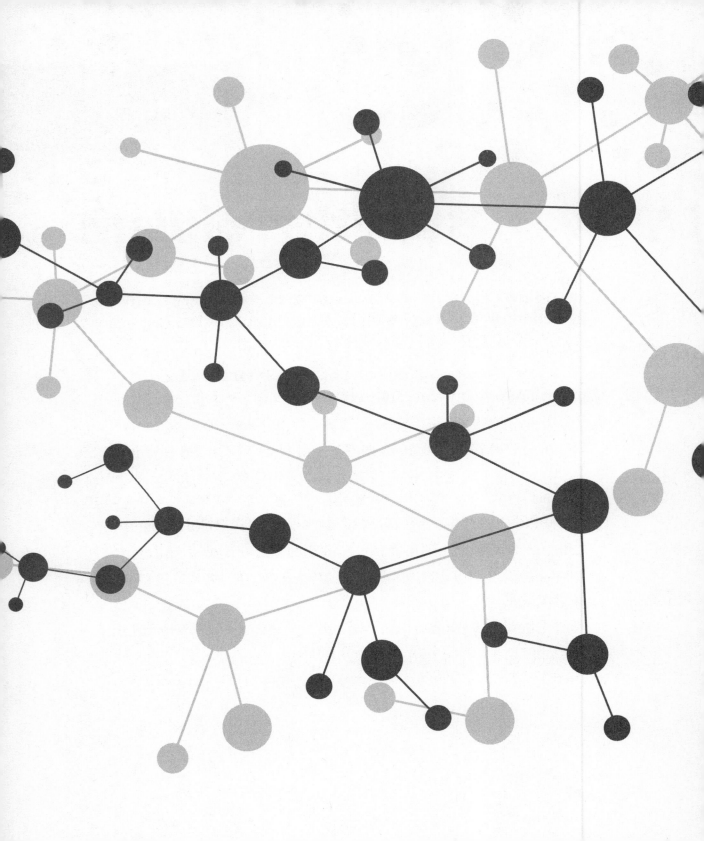

Types of Hypothyroidism

If you're gaining weight, feeling fatigued, losing hair, becoming depressed, or experiencing any of dozens of other symptoms, you might be *hypothyroid*. Hypothyroidism accounts for four out of five cases of thyroid disease. More than 24 million Americans are estimated to have hypothyroidism, and hundreds of millions of people suffer from it worldwide.

What Is Hypothyroidism?

As explained in Chapter 1, your thyroid regulates the energy level of every cell in your body through the production of its hormones. Hypothyroidism occurs when the levels of those hormones—primarily T3 and T4—are below normal. In fact, the first part of this disease's name, *hypo*, is Greek for *below* (just as *hypo*dermic refers to injections below the skin).

The lack of hormones reduces the activity and regeneration of cells throughout your body. This lowered metabolism can result in dramatic weight gain, sluggishness, confusion, insomnia, lowered sex drive, dry nails and skin, feeling cold, and/or myriad other problems. (For a more complete list, see Chapter 6.)

Hypothyroidism can range from mild thyroid underperformance—resulting in symptoms so subtle you don't consciously notice them—to a total shutdown of your thyroid. You can even be hypothyroid if your thyroid is healthy. For example, a defective pituitary gland can order your thyroid to underperform (as we'll explain shortly), or T3 can be blocked from "powering up" your cells by ailing adrenal glands (see Chapter 14).

Hypothyroidism is a complicated disease. On the one hand, it's easy to treat because inexpensive prescription medication will very effectively replace whatever thyroid hormones you lack.

On the other hand, hypothyroidism is often difficult to recognize because its group of wildly diverse symptoms can seem to have nothing to do with each other. Even experienced doctors who don't happen to be thyroid experts often fail to properly diagnose it. The American Association of Clinical Endocrinologists (AACE) estimates that half of those with hypothyroidism don't know it—making this wide-spread disease a quiet epidemic.

Adding to the problem is the fact most doctors are taught in medical school to prescribe T4-only medication across the board. However, many patients require a mix of T4 and T3 to fully resolve their symptoms. Further, even if you're taking the right medication, it can be tricky to arrive at the precise dosage for achieving optimum health.

This is the first of five chapters providing you with the knowledge you need to meet the various challenges posed by hypothyroidism. Once you've read these chapters, you'll know whether you should see a doctor and how to make sure you receive the best testing, diagnosis, and treatment.

Hashimoto's Disease

Roughly 75–85 percent of hypothyroidism results from *Hashimoto's disease,* a condition in which the thyroid undergoes attacks that damage it and reduce its ability to function.

This illness is named after Hakaru Hashimoto, a Japanese doctor who, in 1912, published a medical analysis of the condition.

Hashimoto's disease strikes women more than five times as often as men, and the odds of getting it increase as you grow older.

Causes of Hashimoto's Disease

Hashimoto's is considered an autoimmune disease. The medical community believes it occurs when your immune system—which normally protects you by attacking foreign invaders such as viruses and bacteria—mistakes your thyroid as a danger and starts attacking it, too.

While no one is certain what causes Hashimoto's, recent studies indicate it might be the result of too much iodine.

It used to be that the primary cause of hypothyroidism was *not enough* iodine, and that's still the case in certain underdeveloped countries. But over the past century, countries such as the United States made major efforts to eliminate iodine deficiency. And those efforts may have gone too far.

For example, in most cases, the safe range for daily iodine intake is 50–199 mcg. But a U.S. FDA study estimates average iodine intake in America—not counting the use of iodized salt—is 138–353 mcg. Adding in a gram of iodized salt raises the average to 183–398 mcg daily. The high end of that range is twice the amount of iodine we should consume. If that doesn't seem like a big deal, see Chapter 18 to learn more... including how reducing iodine intake might reverse Hashimoto's.

Another potential cause of Hashimoto's is a buildup of toxic environmental chemicals in the thyroid.

Your thyroid is especially sensitive to chemicals because it's designed to sift through your blood, and suck in and store even the tiniest amounts of iodine it finds. This ability of your thyroid is normally wonderful, because it means you need to consume only a little bit of iodine for your thyroid to have enough of it to make its hormones.

The problem is that over the last 100 years, our world has become flooded with chemicals. According to the U.S. Environmental Protection Agency, there are more than 100,000 chemicals in commercial use, and over 2,300 new ones are submitted to the EPA for approval every year.

Some of these substances are designed to be toxic—for example, the pesticides used to keep insects away from crops. Others include cheap and mildly toxic substances in products that aren't eaten, but nonetheless get through your skin and into your bloodstream. (This happens a lot with cosmetics.) Yet others become toxic as a processing side effect, such as the corn syrup that some factories make using mercury-based components. Recent testing has found that this results in small amounts of mercury turning up in thousands of snacks and beverages.

The amount of any commercial chemical you're exposed to is supposed to be small enough to be safe, but many of these substances haven't been around long enough for us to know what their long-term effects will be. Just as importantly, no one knows how you'll be affected by the combination of hundreds of chemicals in your daily life that have never been tested together.

This is relevant to your thyroid because the same mechanism that allows it to draw in and store tiny amounts of iodine from your bloodstream also leads it to extract and store toxins you consume that happen to be chemically similar to iodine. The latter include mercury (which is poisonous) and perchlorate (which is used in such products as rocket fuel, and is often present in low-quality drinking water).

The iodine in your thyroid eventually gets used up in the production of hormones, but the toxins don't. So even though your thyroid is taking in very small quantities of toxins, they'll accumulate decade after decade. This means the longer you live, the more likely the toxins you're exposed to will accumulate to serious levels...which is why the risk of developing Hashimoto's increases with age.

The medical community believes that at some point the amount of toxins in your thyroid can become so significant that they'll trigger your body's immune system. Your antibodies (specifically, *thyroid peroxidase* and/or *thyroglobulin* antibodies) will designate them as unwelcome invaders, and multiply to assault the cells containing them and flush them out of your system.

Unfortunately, what often happens is the antibodies will mistake your healthy thyroid cells as being a threat along with the cells harboring toxins. The antibodies will respond by attacking your whole thyroid, and there's no easy way to stop them. (Your doctor could shut down your immune system, but that would be a "cure" worse than the threat to your thyroid.)

However, you might be able to mitigate the disease, or even reverse it, by eliminating the substances causing it. For more about this, see Chapters 18 and 20.

Another potential trigger for Hashimoto's is a respiratory infection that induces your body to create numerous antibodies to combat it. Sometimes, antibodies looking for invaders in your neck will become confused and end up attacking your thyroid—which will begin the chain of events leading to Hashimoto's.

There's also a school of thought that suggests Hashimoto's can be caused by a virus that feeds on toxins, periodically attacks the thyroid, and evades the antibodies sent to kill it. There's a pleasing simplicity to this theory because it doesn't involve your immune system attacking your body; you're just dealing with an unusually hard-to-detect invader with its own agenda. It also fits with the eating changes we recommend in Chapter 18, because while that diet reduces your iodine intake, it simultaneously cuts out virtually all foods likely to have toxic elements that might feed the virus, such as antibiotics, GMO, and lab-born chemicals. So far, there's no medical evidence supporting this theory. But if it makes you feel better to think of your thyroid as being attacked by a virus instead of your own immune system, there's no harm to it as long as it doesn't negatively affect your treatment.

Effects of Hashimoto's Disease

The effects of chronic Hashimoto's assaults vary for different people. If you have a mild case, the disease might reduce your thyroid's ability to produce hormones by around 5 percent a year. In this situation the symptoms are so subtle and gradual that you might not realize you're sick for a long time. But once you begin taking thyroid medication, the numerous specific improvements you'll experience will make you suddenly aware of all the ways your body had gone wrong.

On the other hand, Hashimoto's might attack your thyroid aggressively. This could lead to you developing symptoms in an abrupt and very noticeable way. It could also lead to one or more *goiters,* which are enlargements of your thyroid.

In addition, Hashimoto's can cause temporary *hyper*thyroidism. While the disease will make you hypothyroid over the long term, in its early stages it kills a lot of healthy thyroid cells. As these cells die, they'll spill out whatever hormones they contained. This can inject surges of T4 and T3 into your bloodstream, and bring about such symptoms of hyperthyroidism as a rapidly beating heart, anxiety, and panic attacks. You can obtain relief from these symptoms by taking medication for hyperthyroidism until this stage of the disease—which is called *Hashitoxicosis*—eventually ends and your Hashimoto's stabilizes into keeping you exclusively hypothyroid.

If Hashimoto's is giving you the worst of both worlds by alternately making you hypothyroid and hyperthyroid, your TSH levels might appear *normal* on blood tests. That's because the underproduction of thyroid hormones will be evened out by the hormone surges caused by slaughtered thyroid cells. It's therefore important that the initial lab testing your doctor orders for you includes antibody tests, which will pick up the presence of Hashimoto's regardless of your TSH levels.

Goitrous Hypothyroidism

A *goiter* is a non-cancerous swelling on your thyroid. Your thyroid can grow one goiter or multiple goiters. This condition isn't really a disease unto itself; it's a side effect of other hypothyroid diseases such as Hashimoto's. Goiters happen when your body's low levels of thyroid hormones cause your pituitary gland to send out increasing amounts of TSH. Because your thyroid can't produce enough hormones to meet the pituitary's demands at its current size, it responds by growing more cells. This is an effective strategy under normal circumstances, but when disease or shortages are at play, it's doomed to failure.

For example, if you're suffering from Hashimoto's, the hostile chemical environment created by antibodies will prevent new thyroid cells from being capable of producing hormones.

And for those suffering from insufficient iodine—which is the most common cause of goiters in certain underdeveloped countries—new cells won't help because the thyroid will still lack the iodine needed to construct T4 and T3 molecules. In such cases, the body will continue to lack thyroid hormones; the pituitary gland will keep yelling at the thyroid to do something about it; and the thyroid will hopelessly keep making its goiters bigger.

If your hypothyroidism is treated in its early stages, any goiters that might have developed will never become large enough to be felt or noticed. Once you go on thyroid medication and your hormone levels return to normal, your pituitary gland will stop overstimulating your thyroid and the goiters will simply stop growing.

However, if you've been hypothyroid for a long time without treatment, then one or more goiters might become large enough to become visible in your neck, and/or to cause you trouble when speaking, breathing, or swallowing.

In fact, the primary value of goiters is to make themselves known in this way, because they provide undeniable evidence that your body has a chronic shortage of thyroid hormones that needs to be addressed.

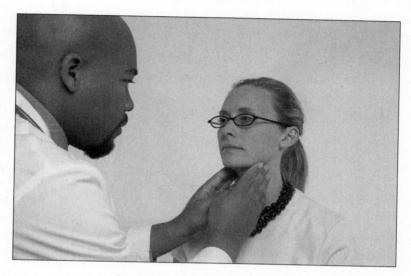

Checking the thyroid for goiters
(Licensed from Shutterstock Images)

Once you're on thyroid medication, your goiters will probably go away over time. Your pituitary gland will not only stop stimulating their growth but will stop encouraging the replacement of dying goiter cells with fresh ones, resulting in natural shrinkage. If your goiters don't disappear on their own, though, and if they're large enough to be uncomfortable and/or cosmetically displeasing, you can opt to have them surgically removed.

It's a good idea to check your neck periodically for growths, which could end up being harmless goiters or—much more rarely—cancer nodules (see Chapter 13). To do so, first get a handheld mirror and a glass of water. Hold the mirror in front of you and, while keeping your eyes focused on the lower portion of your neck, drink the water. If you see any bulges that probably shouldn't be there when you swallow, visit your doctor to have them checked out. However, don't get confused by your Adam's apple; your thyroid is below it, closer to your collarbone.

Pituitary Gland Disease

As explained in Chapter 1, your pituitary gland manages the activity of your thyroid by producing TSH whenever your body needs additional thyroid hormones. Most cases of hypothyroidism result from an ailing thyroid being unable to entirely fulfill the orders represented by the TSH.

However, you can also become hypothyroid if your pituitary gland becomes ill and starts underproducing TSH. In this case, even though your thyroid is entirely healthy, it'll end up making too little T4 and T3 because that's effectively what it's being told to do.

This situation, called *pituitary disease,* can be picked up by standard thyroid blood tests. That's because when you're hypothyroid, you'll normally have low thyroid hormone levels and high TSH levels—the latter being a result of your pituitary gland screaming, "Make more hormones!" If the problem is with your pituitary gland, though, you'll have low hormone levels *and* low TSH.

As a double check, your doctor can test the levels of other hormones regulated by your pituitary gland, such as those produced by your adrenal glands and sex glands. The odds are high that they'll be low as well.

The most common cause for your pituitary malfunctioning is developing a non-cancerous growth called an *adenoma.* If the adenoma is tiny—14 millimeters or less—your doctor will treat it with medication such as *bromocriptine* that can slow, and even reverse, adenoma growth. If the adenoma is larger, though, then its continued growth risks putting dangerous pressure on your nearby optic nerves. In this situation, you should consider surgery to cut out the adenoma.

Therapeutic Hypothyroidism

No matter what type of thyroid disease you start out with, chances are your doctors will cause you to end up hypothyroid. This is called *therapeutic hypothyroidism* because it results from treatment you receive for a thyroid disorder.

For example, if you're hyperthyroid, your treatment might involve surgery or radiation to reduce the size of your thyroid. In a perfect world, the reduction would be so precise that you'd end up with normal hormone production. What's more likely to happen, though, is your doctor will err on the side of making you mildly hypothyroid. That's because you're much safer being hypothyroid than hyperthyroid, and the hypothyroidism can be easily managed with medication.

As another—and more extreme—example, if you have thyroid cancer, you and your doctor might decide to surgically remove your entire thyroid. This will make you hypothyroid because your body will no longer produce any thyroid hormones on its own. Once you start taking thyroid medication, however, your T4 and T3 levels will return to normal.

By far the most common scenario for therapeutic hypothyroidism is being on thyroid medication but remaining somewhat hypothyroid. This can happen if you're exclusively on a T4 prescription when your body happens to also require direct T3. It can also occur if you're taking the right medications but at dosages that are too low. In such cases, trust what you're feeling and observing. If your physician won't acknowledge that you're still hypothyroid, seek a doctor who'll focus on your symptoms instead of just your lab tests (see Chapters 4 and 22).

Drug-Induced Hypothyroidism

While therapeutic hypothyroidism stems from thyroid treatment, *drug-induced hypothyroidism* occurs when you become hypothyroid from medication that has nothing to do with your thyroid.

For example, patients taking lithium—typically for bipolar disorder—have a 50 percent chance of becoming hypothyroid and growing goiters as a side effect of the drug. That's because lithium is chemically similar enough to iodine that the thyroid might eventually start pulling it from the bloodstream and storing it, not leaving enough room for the thyroid to store adequate amounts of iodine. It's largely for this reason that lithium is no longer a doctor's first choice. However, it's still prescribed when other medications don't work.

An even more problematic drug is *amiodarone*, which is used to stabilize an irregular heartbeat. Amiodarone has severe side effects, with hypothyroidism being among the milder ones.

As a rule, whenever your doctor prescribes a medication with which you aren't familiar, make a point of looking up its side effects, and then pay close attention to your body to see if any of them occur. This can be tricky with hypothyroidism because its symptoms aren't always obvious. When you're in doubt, err on the side of caution and get your blood tested. If it turns out the drug is lowering your hormone levels, switch to another drug if possible, or start taking thyroid medication to make up for its effects.

Toxin-Induced Hypothyroidism

As explained previously, if your thyroid accumulates small amounts of toxins over a long time, it might develop Hashimoto's disease. However, it's also possible to take in a relatively large amount of toxins in a short period of time. If the toxins are chemically like iodine, then you'll become hypothyroid. In addition, you might experience severe symptoms beyond hypothyroidism. If the problem is detected early enough, though, treatment might spare you from any permanent damage.

For example, a patient named Dorothy came to me with pain in her muscles. Dorothy was used to starting a new exercise regime and having several days of muscle pain afterward. That's normal, but Dorothy was now constantly experiencing this kind of pain in almost all her muscles, even without exercising. Accompanying this were severe fatigue, trouble sleeping, and depression. Dorothy was on pain medications and antidepressants, and her quality of life was miserable.

Dorothy tested positive for hypothyroidism, and in addition was found to have high levels of mercury in her blood. She underwent treatment to remove the mercury from her body and begin taking low doses of thyroid medication. Over time, Dorothy felt enormously better and was able to wean herself off all the antidepressant and pain medications. And because the problem was caused by toxins rather than a permanently defective thyroid, Dorothy was eventually able to wean herself off her thyroid medication as well.

Iodine-Induced Hypothyroidism

Some people have the notion that if a reasonable amount of a substance is good for you, then taking a lot of it will be even better. The opposite is usually true, and a prime example is iodine.

Earlier in this chapter, we explained that taking in even small amounts of excess iodine regularly could result in hypothyroidism over time.

So as you might imagine, consuming an exceptionally large amount of iodine is even worse. This can happen if you start taking an over-the-counter thyroid "health" product with an absurdly large amount of iodine, or if you're unlucky enough to have an alternative medicine practitioner who prescribes daily iodine megadoses of 1,000–50,000 mcg. In such cases, your thyroid might react by fully shutting down.

The reason is a flood of iodine risks your thyroid abruptly making way too much of its hormones, a condition called a *thyroid storm*. In turn, this puts you in jeopardy of going into such a severe hyperthyroid state that your heart pounds in your chest until you have a heart attack.

Your body understands this danger, so when you feed it too much iodine it "blows a fuse" and turns your thyroid off. Your thyroid won't start working again until your body flushes the excess iodine from your system over 2–3 weeks.

If you continue pumping extreme doses of iodine into your body day after day, though, you may keep your thyroid shut down long enough to do permanent damage to it.

Alternatively, your antibodies might perceive the excess iodine as a toxic invader and start attacking both it and your thyroid cells. This can lead to Hashimoto's disease; or even worse, Graves' disease (see Chapter 10).

Excess iodine can also lead to growths on your thyroid. Sometimes these will be harmless goiters, but sometimes they end up being cancerous.

The way to avoid all this is simple—stay within the recommended range of 50–199 mcg of iodine a day. That means saying *no* to megadose iodine pills. And it also means being aware of the iodine content of what you consume.

For instance, if you eat a great deal of seafood daily, you might be taking in too much iodine. (In fact, seaside villages tend to have high rates of thyroid disease.)

As another example, if you're on the desiccated thyroid medications Nature-Throid or WP Thyroid, you're taking in 130 mcg of iodine with each 1 grain pill, which is all the supplemental iodine your body requires.

For an effective and healthy way to cut back on iodine, see Chapter 18.

If you're not yet sure whether you have hypothyroidism, the next few chapters will provide you with ways to identify it via symptoms and blood tests; and if you do have it, these chapters will explain your options for treating the disease and fully restoring your health.

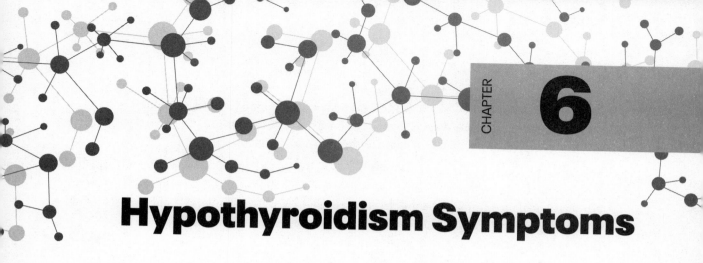

Hypothyroidism Symptoms

I was so exhausted, I couldn't figure out what was going on in my life. I ended up going to Africa and spent a month with my beautiful daughters there, was still feeling tired, really tired, going around from doctor to doctor trying to figure out what was wrong.

—Oprah Winfrey on her hypothyroidism

Hypothyroidism is often hard to identify because it can create any of dozens of seemingly unrelated symptoms, ranging from abrupt weight gain to fatigue to hair loss to depression. Even excellent physicians who don't happen to be thyroid experts might not recognize when you're hypothyroid.

While Chapter 2 covered all thyroid diseases, this chapter focuses squarely on hypothyroidism. It begins with a checklist of symptoms to help you decide if you're hypothyroid. It then provides some real-life stories about patients who thoroughly overcame hypothyroid problems with inexpensive medication.

Once you're done reading, you'll have a checklist of symptoms you can take to your doctor for testing, diagnosis, and possible treatment.

Acknowledging Symptoms

Your thyroid regulates your energy levels by producing hormones that allow your cells to stay "powered up" and active and to grow and generate new cells. Because every part of your body requires energy, if your thyroid starts underproducing these hormones you might experience any number of issues involving your skin, your hair, your brain, your sexual organs, and more.

Some symptoms might be obvious, such as sudden weight gain or severe tiredness. Others might be so subtle—such as feeling confused or less interested in sex—that you're unlikely to immediately recognize them as the results of an illness.

Diagnosing hypothyroidism is tricky for doctors as well. Different patients can have completely different symptoms, combinations of symptoms, and severities of symptoms—all stemming from an off-kilter thyroid. While most hypothyroid issues aren't immediately serious, they can become dangerous over time. And either way, they have a significant negative impact on quality of life.

There are millions of people who suffer with debilitating problems simply because neither they nor their doctors have recognized the root cause as insufficient thyroid hormones. It's a tragedy, because you can easily make up for any lack of T4 and T3 with inexpensive pills...but not until your hypothyroidism has been identified.

> I was depressed, I kept gaining weight, and I had no interest in sex. My doctor sent me to a psychiatrist, but that didn't help at all. Then my hair started falling out.
>
> **—Patient who fully recovered after going on thyroid medication**

Too often, we rationalize changes in our bodies, altering our perceptions of what's normal instead of acknowledging there's something wrong. This chapter will empower you to listen to your body if it's saying your thyroid is underperforming.

Also, keep in mind that if you have a thyroid disorder, you're far from alone. Famous people who've suffered from thyroid disease and thrived after treatment include politicians Hillary Rodham Clinton and Bernie Sanders, hip-hop singer Missy Elliott, pop singer Sia, singer and talk show host Kelly Clarkson, rock stars Linda Ronstadt and Rod Stewart, talk show host Wendy Williams, actresses Gina Rodriguez (star of *Jane the Virgin*) and Sofia Vergara (co-star of *Modern Family* and *America's Got Talent*), tennis player Kiki Bertens, fitness guru Jillian Michaels, and supermodel Gigi Hadid.

Hypothyroidism Symptoms Checklist

Because thyroid hormones affect every cell, in theory, an underactive thyroid can result in any of hundreds of symptoms. In general, though, certain symptoms are more likely to occur than others. These frequent clues to hypothyroidism appear in the checklist that follows.

Take a few minutes to go over the list, and check off any symptom that applies to you. If you aren't sure whether you have a symptom, find the description of it in Chapter 2, and also see if it's covered in the patient stories that follow. Use that additional information to make your decision.

Hypothyroidism Symptoms Checklist

- O Gaining weight for no apparent reason
- O Frequent exhaustion
- O Sluggishness
- O Slowed thinking
- O Memory problems
- O Depression
- O Lowered interest in sex
- O Menstrual problems
- O Infertility
- O Insomnia
- O Constipation
- O Hair loss
- O Thinning or dry hair

- O Dry, brittle nails
- O Rough, itchy, and/or thinning skin
- O Acne
- O Puffy skin
- O Cold skin
- O Feeling unusually cold
- O Sweating too little
- O Numbness in the hands and feet
- O Weak muscles
- O Hoarse voice
- O Enlarged neck

If you have six or more of these common symptoms, there's a strong chance you're hypothyroid. Get your thyroid checked out—typically via blood tests for TSH, free T4, free T3, and antibodies—as soon as possible.

If you have two to five of these symptoms, that's still reason enough to get your thyroid tested. Either the results will be positive, putting you on the path to treatment, or they'll be negative, which will inform your doctor to explore other potential problem sources. (Before accepting a negative result, though, see Chapter 7.)

But even if you have only one of these symptoms and your doctor isn't providing a satisfying explanation for its cause, you should seriously consider getting tested. That's especially true if you're a woman 30 to 50 years old, as that's the gender and age range most often struck by hypothyroidism.

The checklist is by no means comprehensive; you can experience other symptoms. However, the odds are that along with the unlisted symptoms you'll have at least a few of the ones on the checklist.

If you're successfully treated, you'll soon experience improvement regarding *all* your hypothyroidism symptoms.

Hypothyroid Patient Stories

It's easier to understand symptoms when they're viewed within the context of people's lives. The following are true stories of people struggling with medical problems that turned out to be the results of hypothyroidism. Most of these patients had been misdiagnosed before they turned to me for help. They were all restored to full health via inexpensive thyroid medication.

Memory Problems

JoAnne was a delightful woman in her early 70s who abruptly began suffering from impaired mental functioning. JoAnne used to enjoy moderating Civil War discussion groups and traveling to historic battlegrounds, but her memory suddenly became so poor that she gave up all such activities. JoAnne's children were concerned she was experiencing dementia or early Alzheimer's, and had made an appointment for her to see a neurologist. She came to me first in hopes of discovering a more treatable cause.

When I started asking JoAnne questions, it became clear that she wasn't only losing her memory, she was losing her enthusiasm for life. She told me her best friend had switched from calling her a "spitfire" to calling her an "old dishrag." That made JoAnne a prime candidate for thyroid testing.

JoAnne proved to be very clearly hypothyroid. Medication quickly turned things around.

It's fortunate we caught the problem relatively early. In cases where memory loss lasts for more than 18 months, full function often doesn't return even after treatment.

Fatigue and Depression (and Why Symptoms Trump Labs)

Susan was a kind woman under my care for chronic fatigue syndrome. The most prominent aspect of her illness was a dark, foreboding depression. After she grew to trust me, Susan described how the depression felt in painful detail. She then added she saw no reason to subject others to it, so she put on a "public face" when she was with family and friends. I deeply wanted to cure her, but months went by with no significant progress.

One day Susan mentioned reading that depression was sometimes caused by hypo-thyroidism. "Thyroid disease was one of the first things I tested for," I said, "but your lab results showed nothing unusual. If you're willing to risk temporary hyper-thyroid side effects, though, I can give you a low dose of thyroid hormones to see whether they do any good." Susan agreed; and to my surprise, the medication made a substantial improvement in how she felt. I was also surprised that Susan's next series of blood tests showed no significant change in her thyroid hormone levels.

I ended up increasing Susan's dosage four times before her levels clearly went up; and when they did, they were still within the "normal" range. Susan was a perfect example of a patient for whom the numbers didn't tell the whole story.

After a couple of months on the medication, Susan's fatigue and depression entirely lifted. Susan responded by happily throwing away her antidepressant drugs...which had never helped her because they didn't address her real problem, which was hidden hypothyroidism.

This story illustrates a key point. While this chapter is about testing, the fact is too many doctors focus exclusively on numbers. A diagnosis must be a balance of lab results and symptoms—and when in doubt, favor symptoms.

Fatigue and Brittle Nails

Jason was a professional flamenco guitarist who normally loved his job, but over the past year, he had lost his motivation to compose and perform music. He rationalized his lack of energy as career burnout and old age—but he was only in his late 20s!

When I started questioning Jason, he casually mentioned that his fingernails had become a problem. His style of guitar playing depends on long, well-manicured nails. But at around the same time his enthusiasm went downhill, his nails became brittle and kept breaking when picking guitar strings. Jason's manicurist applied increasingly greater levels of protectant, but it didn't help. To be thorough, I tested Jason's zinc and protein levels as well as his thyroid levels. The lab results clearly showed hypothyroidism.

After a year of treatment, Jason's nails were in top shape again. And more importantly, his passion for music and performing had been completely restored.

Feeling Unusually Cold

Caroline came to see me in the middle of the summer wearing heavy pants and a very heavy sweater. When we shook hands, I felt that she was freezing. When I mentioned this, she replied, "All offices keep their temperatures much lower than they ought to." She added, "My husband tries to do the same thing at home, but I won't let him."

Caroline was already taking thyroid medication, but on a low dosage. I gradually raised it, and after a few months Caroline was dressing normally and enjoying warmth again.

Hair Loss

One of the symptoms that most strongly motivates people to see me without delay is hair loss. Sally was a patient of mine for years and had been treated successfully for her hypothyroidism. One day Sally came to see me in a panic. She leaned her head forward and showed me the clear thinning of her hair, with lots of scalp showing.

"We need to raise my thyroid medication right away!" Sally said.

"It could be your thyroid," I replied, "but it could be something else. Let me take your blood and have the lab test for the likeliest causes."

The results showed Sally's instincts were right. She tested negative for everything except her previous problem—she'd again become hypothyroid.

I was puzzled because Sally's condition had been stable for years. I asked if she was taking her medication first thing in the morning, and was waiting 30–60 minutes before eating or drinking anything but water. She assured me she was.

I increased Sally's dosage, expecting her thyroid hormone levels to rise on her next test. A month later, I received another surprise: the levels had gotten even *lower*.

The situation had become so unusual that I decided to question Sally more carefully about her morning routine. This time she mentioned that a few months ago she'd begun taking her thyroid pills with orange juice instead of water. "But that shouldn't make any difference," she added.

"Is it calcium-fortified orange juice?" I asked.

"Yes, it is," she replied.

I shook my head. "Sally, calcium is one of the strongest binders of thyroid hormones. You aren't giving the hormones a chance to get into your bloodstream."

I put Sally back on her original dosage and asked her to take her medication with water only. Sally's blood levels quickly returned to normal, and within a few months over 90 percent of her hair had grown back.

Infertility

Monica was a 30-year-old who'd tried for years to conceive, with no success. In such cases, low progesterone is often the culprit. When I spoke to Monica, however, I learned that she'd been gaining weight over the past few years. She'd chalked it up to "growing older."

I tested Monica's blood, and she turned out to be hypothyroid. This should've been picked up by Monica's gynecologist or fertility specialist, but it never occurred to either of them to check her for thyroid disease.

As it turned out, Monica was quite fertile. Within two months of starting on thyroid medication, she became pregnant. A few years later, my wife and I ran into Monica and her two children—the second was conceived shortly after the first was born. Monica proudly showed off her new family and thanked me exuberantly. My wife mentioned friends of hers who I'd also treated successfully for infertility, adding, "Oh yeah, he gets everybody pregnant!" I was quite embarrassed, but the two of them had a good laugh over it.

Muscle Weakness

Janet was diagnosed with debilitating fibromyalgia syndrome when she was 16. She'd been forced to drop out of school because of her unremitting muscle pain and weakness. She needed her mother's help with such simple things as getting out of bed and dressing. Janet had seen a mob of doctors—rheumatologists, neurologists, and alternative practitioners. They all said her problem was exclusively fibromyalgia syndrome.

Three years later, at age 19, Janet came to see me. The tests I ran showed signs of an old Epstein-Barr viral respiratory infection, thyroid antibodies, and a TSH that was above normal levels. Apparently, Janet developed Hashimoto's as a result of her respiratory infection at age 16...and had been hypothyroid ever since.

After six months of thyroid medication, Janet regained over 80 percent of her muscular strength, and her pain all but disappeared. I prescribed exercises for her to perform to get the rest of the strength back in her arms and legs.

Similar and Overlapping Conditions

If you're experiencing hypothyroid symptoms, you shouldn't hesitate to see a doctor and get your blood tested for TSH, free T4, free T3, and thyroid antibodies. However, that doesn't mean you should skip other types of testing.

There are conditions that cause many of the same symptoms as hypothyroidism, and it's possible that your problems are stemming from one of them. Further, it's possible that you're suffering from hypothyroidism and some other condition *simultaneously*. Certain conditions not only resemble but frequently coexist with hypothyroidism, making normally unpleasant symptoms even worse. For much more about this, see Chapters 17 and 21.

Now that you've identified your symptoms, you're ready to see your doctor to get tested and diagnosed. This is covered next.

Diagnosing Hypothyroidism

If you're experiencing one or more of the symptoms described in Chapter 6 and believe the cause might be hypothyroidism, you shouldn't hesitate to see a doctor and get tested. The initial phase of this process is straightforward—your doctor takes some of your blood, and then sends it to a lab with instructions on which tests to run. What makes things complicated is that many doctors fail to ask for the right combination of tests, and many doctors also fail to correctly interpret the results.

This chapter guides you through the hypothyroidism testing and analysis process. It tells you the best methods for diagnosing your condition, and explains the most common ways in which doctors get important details wrong.

Some physicians dislike patients learning about diagnostic procedures, claiming "A little knowledge is a dangerous thing." But when it comes to hypothyroidism, it's much more dangerous to be uninformed. After reading this chapter you'll know what errors to keep an eye out for, and how to ensure you're receiving the most accurate diagnosis possible.

Key Blood Tests for Hypothyroidism

The perfect way to detect thyroid disease would be to measure how T3 is affecting the energy levels of your cells' "batteries," called mitochondria. If your mitochondria turned out to be low on power, that would be definitive proof you're hypothyroid.

Unfortunately, medical science currently can't check your energy at the cellular level. So instead of one straightforward test, a doctor who's a thyroid expert will order four indirect tests: TSH, free T4, free T3, and thyroid antibodies. No single test tells the whole story. But if a doctor is experienced at analyzing the results from all of these tests combined—while at the same time paying attention to your symptoms—the chances are great that she'll be able to judge both whether you're hypothyroid and what sort of treatment you need.

If you're already on thyroid medication, and/or if you're taking other prescription medications or over-the-counter supplements, schedule your doctor's appointment for the morning and delay taking your pills until after your blood's been extracted. This will decrease the chances of anything skewing your test results.

TSH

Your thyroid increases and decreases its hormone production based on the orders it receives from a small organ just above your sinuses called the pituitary gland. When your body is low on energy, your pituitary gland responds by making thyroid stimulating hormone (TSH). As its name indicates, TSH stimulates your thyroid, effectively telling it, "We need more power. Get to work and produce more hormones."

Labs can detect the level of TSH in your bloodstream. When your TSH is above normal, it means you don't have enough thyroid hormones, and in response your pituitary gland is releasing more TSH than usual to tell your thyroid to step up production. Conversely, if your TSH is below normal, it means your thyroid hormone level is too high, and in response your pituitary gland is releasing less TSH than usual to slow your thyroid's production. In other words, there's an inverse relationship between your TSH and thyroid hormone levels because your pituitary gland is continually trying to address any imbalance.

At first blush, it might seem that the TSH test will tell you everything you need to know. In fact, many doctors mistakenly order this test exclusively to check on your thyroid. But relying on the TSH alone is a serious mistake.

First, the TSH level in your bloodstream isn't a snapshot of your current condition. Instead, it represents a 2–3 month average of your pituitary gland's activities. That's good in that it provides a long-term look at your body. However, it means you can experience hypothyroid symptoms for some time before your condition is fully reflected by the TSH test. This can lead to a doctor pronouncing "you're normal" when you're really in the early stages of hypothyroidism.

Further, if you have Hashimoto's disease, you might swing back and forth between hypothyroidism and hyperthyroidism, a condition called Hashitoxicosis. Because the TSH is a long-term average, the two extremes can cancel each other out, resulting in a TSH level that's normal...and that's masking the war occurring between your immune system and your thyroid.

In addition, the TSH level doesn't reflect whether your thyroid hormones are successfully energizing your cells. For example, if you have plenty of T4 but it's not being converted to T3 (see Chapter 1), or if your T3 can't penetrate your cells (see Chapter 14), your TSH level will be normal but you'll be hypothyroid.

Then again, you could have a healthy thyroid but an ailing pituitary gland. For example, if your pituitary is underactive, it'll cause your thyroid to underproduce hormones; but the low TSH level will make your doctor think that you have the opposite problem and are hyperthyroid.

So while the TSH test is a very useful tool, it's not enough by itself to evaluate your status.

On the flip side of the coin, you might hear advocates of old-school thyroid methods claim the TSH test is inaccurate. It's true that a doctor relying on the TSH test alone will reach incorrect conclusions for a substantial number of patients. But all this means is your doctor should run a TSH test in conjunction with other key thyroid tests—and while carefully considering your symptoms—to paint a complete picture. To abandon TSH testing as old-school disciples recommend would be throwing away one of the most helpful diagnostic tools available for your health.

Free T4 and Free T3

As explained in Chapter 1, roughly 85–90 percent of the hormones made by your thyroid are T4. T4 is a "storage" hormone designed to circulate in your bloodstream, and be stored in your tissues, until thyroid hormone is needed by an area of your body. When energy is called for, your body converts T4 to T3. And it's T3 that does the work of powering up the mitochondria in your cells.

Labs can easily measure the amount of T4 in your bloodstream that's available for conversion, which is called *free T4*. And labs can also easily measure the amount of your circulating T3 that's available for your body's immediate use, which is called *free T3*.

Unlike the TSH test that reflects a 2–3 month average, the free T4 and free T3 tests reflect the activities of those hormones within the past week or so. These tests offer a more immediate picture of what's happening in your body.

If you're wondering what makes these versions of T4 and T3 "free:" Your body renders more than 96 percent of T3 and over 99 percent of T4 molecules inert by binding them with proteins. (No one knows why, though some speculate it's a way of preserving iodine beyond what can be stored in the thyroid.) However, it's only the unbound, or "free," hormones that have any effect on your health. Free T4 and free T3 can't be accurately calculated from total T4/T3, because there are a variety of factors that can affect the totals (ranging from pregnancy to how much protein you've recently eaten) but have no impact on the free hormones. So be wary of any doctor who runs old-fashioned total T4/T3 tests instead of modern free T4/T3 tests.

Evaluating your TSH level in conjunction with free T4 and free T3 levels provides a much clearer view than can be gotten from considering TSH alone. For example, if you're in the early stages of hypothyroidism, the 2–3 month average represented by your TSH level might not reflect the recent changes in your body; but the more "in the moment" free T4/T3 numbers will show up as low, alerting your doctor to the problem. Catching hypothyroidism early gives you the opportunity to go on a low dosage of medication while trying the dietary changes recommended in Chapter 18—and possibly stop the disease in its tracks.

As another example, if your pituitary gland is underactive, your TSH level will be low, making you appear hyperthyroid. However, if your free T4/T3 is *also* low, an experienced thyroid doctor will know to suspect a pituitary problem and prescribe an ultrasound or MRI to take a close look at that gland.

Then again, your body might be having trouble converting T4 into T3. A frequent cause of this is a lack of selenium, which can be cured by simply eating a Brazil nut a day. (Don't eat more than one a day regularly, as that could eventually result in an overdose.) If conversion is the issue, your TSH and your free T4 levels will both be normal, but your free T3 level will be low.

The latter is a perfect example of why it's important to test for free T4 *and* free T3. Many doctors are knowledgeable enough to order TSH and free T4 tests, but then neglect to include the free T3 test. These doctors assume that the free T3 level will merely echo the level of free T4. While they'll be correct most of the time, in my experience 20–30 percent of hypothyroid patients will have a discrepancy between their T4 and T3 levels. More specifically, these patients' T4 levels will be proportionally higher than their T3 levels, indicating conversion problems. If you happen to be one of these patients, you're at risk of being prescribed the wrong treatment when free T3 testing is skipped.

If your doctor tests your blood for TSH, free T4, and free T3, the results will provide a pretty good view of your thyroid's status. However, there's one other test category needed to complete the picture.

Antibodies

As mentioned previously, the early stages of Hashimoto's disease—which is the cause of roughly 75–85 percent of hypothyroidism cases—can create a condition of Hashitoxicosis in which you're swinging between levels of thyroid hormones that are too low and too high. The two extremes can cancel each other out, resulting in a TSH level that appears normal. At the same time, your free T4/T3 levels will depend on the state of your Hashitoxicosis over the week before you happen to have your blood taken. In other words, they might be low, high, or even normal, depending on what stage of the pendulum swing the disease is in.

Therefore, when you're first being diagnosed, it's important to test for thyroid antibodies. More specifically, your doctor should test for *thyroid peroxidase* (*TPO*) antibodies and *thyroglobulin* (*Tg*) antibodies. If you have Hashimoto's, the chances are you'll have high levels of one or both antibodies.

That said, thyroid antibody testing is only required for your initial diagnosis. For your follow-up visits, your doctor needs to order just the TSH, free T4, and free T3 tests.

Other Testing

Even if your symptoms point strongly to hypothyroidism, you shouldn't hesitate to allow your doctor to test for other causes. It's possible some other disease is responsible. And it's just as possible that you're hypothyroid and have another condition occurring at the same time, making your life doubly difficult (see Chapter 21).

In addition, you might require examination that goes beyond blood tests. For example, if your doctor suspects you have Hashimoto's disease based on your symptoms but it's not showing up in the lab numbers, he might prescribe an ultrasound to check for evidence of cellular destruction.

Alternatively, if your doctor notices a growth on your thyroid during your physical exam, you might require ultrasound testing, and possibly a biopsy, to determine whether the growth is dangerous (see Chapter 13).

Regardless of the results from the lab, always pay attention to your symptoms. If your body is sending you messages and your test results don't reflect them, then the problem is usually with the testing, not with what you're feeling.

Analyzing Your Test Results

A few days after your doctor sends your blood to a lab, the test results—which are typically a small collection of numbers fitting onto a single sheet of paper—will be transmitted to her office. As explained in Chapter 4, you can request that her office email or fax that same one-page report to you. You can then study the results at your leisure before the next visit to your doctor. This will allow you to know what to expect, and to prepare any pertinent questions.

Alternatively, you can request a photocopy of the results be mailed to you, or you can pick it up at your doctor's office. Being able to see the precise numbers will empower you to know exactly where you're at, help you more clearly understand how your doctor arrived at her diagnosis, and allow you to double-check your doctor's conclusions.

When you receive test results, first check to make sure they include your correct name and birthdate. Both labs and doctors' offices handle thousands of patients, and mistakes happen.

Each of your tests will result in a single number that's judged by where it falls within the range considered normal for that test. The key thyroid tests and their ranges are as follows:

Key Tests and Ranges for Hypothyroidism

Test name	Typical lab range	Optimal range
TSH	0.4–4.5 mIU/L	0.3–2.0 mIU/L
Free T4	0.8–1.8 ng/dL	1.1–1.8 ng/dL
Free T3	230–420 pg/dL	same as lab
Thyroid Peroxidase (TPO) Antibodies	<35 IU/mL	same as lab
Thyroglobulin (Tg) Antibodies	<20 IU/mL	same as lab

Interpreting results using these ranges is mostly straightforward. For example, if your free T3 level is 300 *pg/dL* (*picograms per deciliter* of blood), then it's normal because it falls within the range of 230–420 pg/dL. Alternatively, if your T3 level is 50 pg/dL, then it's much too low and you're probably hypothyroid.

Similarly, if either of your antibody counts is 900 IU/mL (*international unit for antibodies per milliliter* of blood), that's way over the normal limit—35 for TPO and 20 for Tg—and indicates your thyroid is under attack.

Interpreting TSH and free T4 lab test results can sometimes be more complicated, though. That's because there's a discrepancy between the recommended range used by most labs and what thyroid experts believe is the actual optimal range for good health. If your results fall within the narrower ranges recommended by the experts, then they're also within a typical lab's range, and your diagnosis is straightforward. But if your results happen to fall into the gray area between your lab's ranges and the optimal ranges, then the next section is of vital importance to you.

Why "Normal" Results Might Be Wrong

This chapter previously described how your doctor might pronounce you healthy if he relied on too few blood tests (such as TSH alone, or TSH and free T4 alone). But your doctor might also misdiagnose you as being fine because your results are all in the "normal" range. It's not that the test results are wrong. Labs usually provide highly accurate measurements. The problem is with the ranges used by the labs for what's considered "normal." For TSH, most labs use a broad range of 0.4–4.5 mIU/L (milli-international units per liter of blood). Some labs use an even higher upper limit than 4.5 mIU/L, such as 5.0, 5.5, or a jaw-dropping 6.0.

These ranges were created by averaging the results of numerous people who've been tested. That's a technique that often works; but for reasons that are still being debated, it doesn't work for the TSH test. Based on real-world experience, most thyroid experts consider the real range for TSH to be much narrower.

The American Association of Clinical Endocrinologists (AACE) recommends using a TSH range of 0.3–3.0 mIU/L. And based on my own clinical experience with tens of thousands of thyroid patients, I use an even narrower range of 0.3–2.0 mIU/L. Studies have shown this is the range that results when testing only people who have no thyroid disease (as opposed to lab averages mostly comprised of patients with hypothyroid symptoms). Why shouldn't you be compared to the healthy?

There's a similar, although less extreme, situation for free T4. Most labs use a range of 0.8–1.8 ng/dL (nanograms per deciliter of blood). In my experience, more accurate is the narrower range of 1.1–1.8 ng/dL.

In other words, if a patient with pertinent symptoms has a TSH level a bit above 2.0 mIU/L, and it's coupled with a free T4 level a bit below 1.1 ng/dL, I'll treat that patient for mild hypothyroidism. In most cases, the patient will improve within a few weeks of being on thyroid medication. Unfortunately, this scenario is more the exception than the rule. When a lab puts a test result in the "normal" column, most busy doctors will simply accept it, favoring hard numbers over a patient's symptoms.

To put it more concretely: Labs lay out their reports by setting results deemed ordinary in plain type, and the results considered to be unusual in boldface or highlighted in gray. This draws a busy doctor's eye away from anything designated In Range. Doctors joke that WNL, or Within Normal Limits, really stands for We Never Looked. But it's a genuinely serious problem if a lab's use of a range that's too broad causes your hypothyroidism to be ignored.

It's been estimated that tens of millions of people are unknowingly suffering from hypothyroidism. It's bad enough that many of them don't understand the disease sufficiently to identify its symptoms; and still worse that many of the ones who seek help are let down by doctors who *also* fail to recognize hypothyroidism symptoms. But it's downright tragic when a patient suspects hypothyroidism, sees a doctor to get tested for it...and is told she's "normal" because her TSH level isn't above the lab's excessive upper range.

Don't let this happen to you. If your test results happen to fall into the gray area between lab ranges and what thyroid experts know to be a more accurate range, discuss the AACE's recommended range of 0.3–3.0 mIU/L—and this book's recommended upper limit of 2.0—with your doctor. If your symptoms persist, and your doctor refuses to treat you with thyroid medication, then use Chapter 4, Chapter 22, and Appendix B to find a different doctor.

Analyzing Patient Test Results

Understanding how to analyze your own test results can be easier after examining real-life examples. The following are true stories of people who were tested for hypothyroidism and, thanks to their being given the right combination of tests and the right interpretation of the results, were successfully diagnosed and treated.

For each patient, you'll see the test results first. Try to analyze the numbers, and then read the patient's tale to find out if you've interpreted them correctly.

Memory Problems

Test name	In range	Out of range	Lab range	Optimal range
TSH		24.65 mIU/L	0.4-4.5 mIU/L	0.3-2.0 mIU/L
Free T4		0.5 ng/dL	0.8-1.8 ng/dL	1.1-1.8 ng/dL
Free T3		190 pg/dL	230-420 pg/dL	same as lab
TPO Antibodies		>1,000 IU/mL	<35 IU/mL	same as lab
Tg Antibodies		699 IU/mL	<20 IU/mL	same as lab

Dora came to see me when she was about to flunk out of nursing school. Dora never had academic problems before, but suddenly was finding it impossible to remember what she was reading. She asked if I could recommend any natural memory enhancers. I told her there were lifestyle changes and supplements that could help, but first we should conduct a few simple tests to make sure there were no medical causes for these "out of the blue" symptoms. Dora was skeptical but agreed to humor me.

I doubted the issue was thyroid disease because Dora's only symptom was poor memory, but included thyroid tests to be thorough. As you can see from Dora's results, both her free T4 and free T3 were well below their optimal ranges, and her TSH and antibody counts were through the roof. It was a classic advanced case of Hashimoto's disease.

After seeing these numbers, I was certain Dora's memory problems would disappear once she was on thyroid medication. However, I warned her it could be several months until the mental damage was fully repaired. Happily, Dora's usual excellent memory returned in only a few weeks, and she ended up doing well in all her classes.

Quest for Growth

Test name	In range	Out of range	Lab range	Optimal range
TSH		11.0 mIU/L	0.4-4.5 mIU/L	0.3-2.0 mIU/L
Free T4		0.7 ng/dL	0.8-1.8 ng/dL	1.1-1.8 ng/dL
Free T3		205 pg/dL	230-420 pg/dL	same as lab
TPO Antibodies	11 IU/mL		<35 IU/mL	same as lab
Tg Antibodies	5 IU/mL		<20 IU/mL	same as lab

Bob came to me feeling weak and tired and with a poor libido. A friend of his was taking growth hormone replacement therapy and feeling great, and Bob believed he needed the same thing. "It's not the right treatment for most adults," I told him, "but let's do some tests before making any conclusions." The results showed Bob to be hypothyroid via his low levels of free T4 and T3, and a high TSH of 11. Ironically, other tests showed Bob's growth hormone level was too high as well! When the pituitary gland makes an excessive amount of TSH, it can accidentally release too much growth hormone at the same time. Thyroid medication soon solved all these problems.

Weight Gain

Test name	In range	Out of range	Lab range	Optimal range
TSH	1.5 mIU/L		0.4–4.5 mIU/L	0.3–2.0 mIU/L
Free T4	1.3 ng/dL		0.8–1.8 ng/dL	1.1–1.8 ng/dL
Free T3	320 pg/dL		230–420 pg/dL	same as lab
TPO Antibodies		>1,000 IU/mL	<35 IU/mL	same as lab
Tg Antibodies		77 IU/mL	<20 IU/mL	same as lab

Melody couldn't quite put her finger on it, but she hadn't been feeling "right" for the past six months. She was convinced there was some sort of problem with her body. The final straw was her weight slowly creeping up, even though she was a college student majoring in exercise physiology. In addition, she was feeling anxious for no apparent reason. Melody's family doctor had run some basic blood tests—including ones for TSH and free T4—and then told her she was fine. Not believing him, she came to see me.

Medical schools have a tradition of teaching that patients aren't great judges of their health. However, I've learned that most people have a pretty good sense of what's going on with their bodies. I ordered a more thorough battery of tests for Melody, including those for antibodies. It turned out her thyroid peroxidase (TPO) antibodies were through the roof, and her thyroglobulin (Tg) antibody count was high, too.

Melody's TSH, free T4, and free T3 were all normal. However, the antibodies indicated major trouble was coming unless something was done. I prescribed a very low daily dose of desiccated thyroid, which helped bind up the antibodies and reduce their harmful effects. In addition, I put Mary on the diet in Chapter 18. Over the next few months, Melody's antibody levels substantially decreased. She also lost the extra weight, and her anxiety disappeared.

Depressed but "Normal"

Test name	In range	Out of range	Lab range	Optimal range
TSH	3.7 mIU/L		0.4–4.5 mIU/L	0.3–2.0 mIU/L
Free T4	0.9 ng/dL		0.8–1.8 ng/dL	1.1–1.8 ng/dL

Joan was a 43-year-old mother with a full life who began feeling sad for no apparent reason. Soon after that, Joan became exhausted performing everyday chores that normally gave her no trouble. Joan's normally mild PMS grew severe. She noticed her hair was thinning and she was gaining weight.

Joan went to see her family doctor, who ran TSH and free T4 tests. As you can see, the results were in the lab's "normal" range. Her doctor therefore dismissed Joan's suspicion of thyroid disease and prescribed antidepressants.

Joan felt sure she had a physical problem, so she went to see a different doctor; and then a third doctor. They all told her the same thing: her tests results were "normal."

After Joan gained 30 pounds, a friend of hers recommended me. It took only seconds of looking at her test results to realize Joan was unlucky enough to be in the "gray area" that's within a too-broad lab range but outside the optimal range for health.

I told Joan her symptoms were classic for hypothyroidism, and her TSH and free T4 levels indicated she was in the early stages of the disease. After giving Joan a more complete set of tests—which included antibody testing that showed she had Hashimoto's—I put her on thyroid medication. After several months, all of Joan's symptoms disappeared. Joan then focused on losing the weight she'd gained while doctors were telling her she was fine.

Headaches and Back Pain

Test name	In range	Out of range	Lab range	Optimal range
TSH		0.03 mIU/L	0.4–4.5 mIU/L	0.3–2.0 mIU/L
Free T4		0.6 ng/dL	0.8–1.8 ng/dL	1.1–1.8 ng/dL
Free T3		190 pg/dL	230–420 pg/dL	same as lab
TPO Antibodies	28 IU/mL		<35 IU/mL	same as lab
Tg Antibodies	17 IU/mL		<20 IU/mL	same as lab

Tara had an unusual set of symptoms for a young woman: continual severe head-aches, debilitating back pain, and painful irritable bowel syndrome. She'd already been tested by an internist, a neurologist, a gastroenterologist, and a rheumatologist, but none of them had provided a credible diagnosis or effective treatment. I looked over all her previous tests and saw she'd never been checked for thyroid disease. I therefore ordered basic thyroid testing, along with detailed tests of her bowel function and an MRI of her back.

As you can see, Tara's TSH level was quite low, which by itself is a sign of hyper-thyroidism. However, her free T4 and free T3 levels were also low, which indicated her thyroid gland was underperforming because it was being told to do so by her pituitary gland. Tara's previous doctors had given her a brain MRI, but it didn't provide a good view of her pituitary. I ordered a new MRI that did...and discovered a growth putting so much pressure on her pituitary gland that it prevented full production of TSH and other pituitary hormones.

A pituitary growth that's benign will usually make the same hormones as the gland, leading to excessive TSH. Because that wasn't happening, I suspected cancer. I recommended prompt surgery to remove and identify the growth. The operation went smoothly—and we were all happy to discover the growth *was* benign. Tara's pituitary gland and thyroid quickly returned to normal, so she required no medica-tion; and over the next several months her full health was restored.

Your Always Available Second Opinion

As this chapter has shown, interpreting a lab's thyroid test results correctly involves nuances that many doctors aren't even aware of. We therefore recommend that you make a habit of asking your doctor to provide you with your test results, and that you analyze them yourself using this chapter as your guide.

If your interpretation of the numbers turns out to be different from what your doctor is telling you they mean, discuss it with your doctor to ensure that you receive the treatment you need.

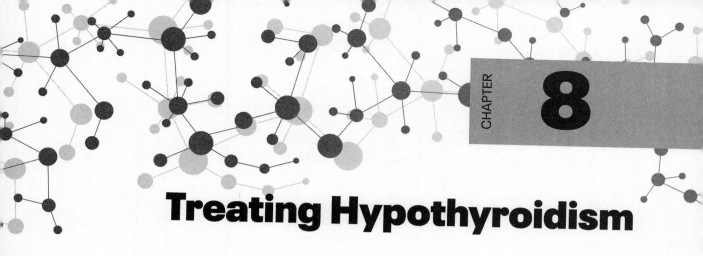

Treating Hypothyroidism

If you've been successfully diagnosed, and your doctor has determined that you're hypothyroid, then you're ready for treatment.

Happily, while hypothyroidism can cause immense suffering until it's addressed, there are few other serious diseases as easy to manage. All you need is thyroid medication, which is inexpensive, relatively harmless, and low maintenance. Taking a pill or two when you wake up each morning will typically do the trick.

Further, you have a number of medications to choose from, ranging from natural to synthetic and from brand name to generic. The key challenge is choosing the medication or combination of medications that most fully meet your needs.

This chapter therefore provides you with extensive information about using medication to treat your hypothyroidism.

Please Note: While most of what follows focuses on prescription medication, you should also read Chapter 18, "Reversing Thyroid Disease Through Diet," and the last section of this chapter for additional approaches we recommend you try in conjunction with taking your thyroid pills.

History of Thyroid Treatment

To understand the options available for thyroid medication, it helps to have some context about the history of thyroid treatment.

Centuries ago, patients with thyroid disease were out of luck. Their doctors were clueless about the cause of their ailments, so their "treatments" were recommendations of warm baths or pleasant environments.

Once doctors figured out that symptoms such as severe lack of energy were caused by an ailing thyroid, they first tried giving patients thyroid tissue as transplants. That made patients feel better...but only for a short time. That's because the tissue was rejected as a transplant, but the patient's body absorbed the tissue and temporarily benefitted from the hormones it contained.

Physicians next tried feeding patients the thyroids of animals, either raw or cooked. This approach was effective, but it was accompanied by serious side effects. Because doctors couldn't tell the level of thyroid hormones in any given gland, there was a lot of guesswork—and a lot of dangerous overdoses. An excessive level of thyroid hormones can cause the heart to beat too fast, potentially resulting in cardiovascular disease and even a heart attack.

Eventually researchers created thyroid medication with a standardized hormonal potency. In the 1890s, crude forms of thyroid extract and natural desiccated thyroid became available. Desiccated thyroid took off, and it became the hypothyroidism treatment of choice for the next 80 years.

The risk of overdosing persisted, though. Doctors based their treatment on patient symptoms, so when issues such as fatigue, weight gain, and confusion improved with more thyroid medication, they tended to prescribe higher doses. But many patients who felt they were doing great on the medication developed heart issues that ended with their early deaths.

The situation improved when physicians realized they could measure basal metabolic rate (BMR) by comparing the amounts of oxygen and carbon dioxide a patient breathed out. (For example, someone with myxedema, a severe form of hypothyroidism, burns energy 40 percent more slowly than normal.) Doctors used the BMR test to both identify thyroid disease and to set a patient's medication dosage to roughly the right level.

But the biggest thyroid testing breakthroughs happened in the 1960s and 1970s. Most notably, researchers found a way of measuring TSH, a hormone from the pituitary gland that tells the thyroid to increase or decrease its production of thyroid hormones. The TSH test provided a reliable way of measuring a body's average thyroid production for the past 2–3 months. And in this same period, researchers developed blood tests that directly measured free T4 and free T3, showing a patient's thyroid hormone status over the past week.

These three tests (in improved forms) are still used today; and when performed together, they give physicians precise ways of seeing what's going on with your thyroid production, both in the long term and short term.

As for thyroid medication, in the 1960s 80 percent of thyroid prescriptions were for natural desiccated thyroid. By then, doctors had the option of prescribing T4-only pills, but they found many patients on T4 felt well only on overdosages that made their TSH dangerously low. This maintained the popularity of desiccated thyroid, which provided both T4 and T3, and tended to make all patients feel well at safe TSH levels.

However, in 1970, it was discovered that most of a person's T3 wasn't produced directly by the thyroid but instead was converted from T4. Doctors no longer assumed it was important to prescribe medication that contained both T4 and T3. They reasoned that T4 was sufficient, because the thyroid would convert the T4 whenever the body needed T3.

In addition, synthetic T4 dosages were precise, while the potency of desiccated thyroid medication at the time was determined by measuring iodine content, which made their T4/T3 levels inconsistent. That was a major mistake, and since 1985 desiccated thyroid manufacturers have switched to measuring the exact amounts of T4 and T3 in their pills, giving them the same precision as synthetic medication.

During the 1970s, though, synthetic thyroid manufacturers used the flaw in that era's desiccated thyroid plus aggressive marketing tactics, to radically change doctors' prescription habits. For example, from 1966 to 1988, natural thyroid prescriptions plummeted from 16.6 million to 4.5 million, while those for synthetic thyroid skyrocketed from 3.6 million to 23.2 million. This apparently irrational bias against medication that provides both T4 and T3 is still taught today in most medical schools, which can make it a challenge to get a prescription for desiccated thyroid from a mainstream doctor.

Modern research paints a different picture, though. Studies have found T4-only medication is effective for many people, but one out of three would have to take dangerous overdoses of T4 to achieve an adequate supply of T3.

Further, even if they have enough T3 in the bloodstream, patients taking only T4 can end up with an inadequate formation of T3 in their tissues.

The straightforward solution to these issues is to take a medication that provides both T4 and T3, such as desiccated thyroid.

Patient Dissatisfaction

Even though the mainstream medical community remains overwhelmingly in favor of T4-only medication, patients feel differently. For example, in 2018 the American Thyroid Association conducted a survey of 12,146 patients, asking what type of treatment they were on, how well they felt their treatment was helping their symptoms, and how satisfied overall they were with treatment. Respondents were 96 percent female, with even age distributions between 31 and 61+. Here are a few highlights:

- More than 33 percent of respondents said they were never given a clear explanation of why they were on thyroid medication.

- Thirty-eight percent were on something other than T4 medication (in most cases, desiccated thyroid). That was a surprise because the ATA itself has advised against this approach. It was expected this number would be under 10 percent.

- Fewer than 7 percent were "very satisfied" with their treatment.

- Issues that continued even after treatment included weight gain, fatigue, mood swings, and memory loss.

- A total of 71 percent of respondents changed doctors multiple times because they weren't satisfied with their thyroid treatment.

- More than 80 percent of respondents expressed a strong need for new treatments of hypothyroidism.

The survey's researchers compared the responses between those on T4 and those on desiccated thyroid. It turned out those on desiccated thyroid were more satisfied with their treatment, and had fewer struggles with weight, fatigue, mood, and memory. As a group, they'd been on thyroid treatment longer and had gone through more doctors.

One of the most compelling findings was the impact thyroid disease had on people's lives. The question was, "How has your life been affected by your hypothyroidism?"

The choice was a number from 1 to 10, with 10 representing the most impact. In all groups, the average answer was 10.

In other words, thyroid disease is having an enormous effect on people's lives...and most of them feel they're being inadequately treated.

Sadly, these survey results are typical. There's increasing evidence the medical community's T4-only approach to thyroid disease is failing far too many people.

How to Take Your Thyroid Medication

Whatever thyroid medication you end up choosing, you should follow certain rules to ensure your meds are fully absorbed.

Most importantly, thyroid medication shouldn't be taken with anything but water. That's because there are numerous foods (ranging from dairy, soy, cabbage, and calcium-enriched juice) and other substances (including iron and calcium) that will bind with the thyroid hormones while they're in your stomach, preventing the hormones from moving on to your small intestine and then to your bloodstream.

You should therefore take your thyroid pill(s) as soon as you wake up in the morning, and wait 30–60 minutes to allow the hormones time to move out of your stomach and into your blood.

You can then eat breakfast and take your vitamins and any other medication.

Desiccated Thyroid

As explained in Chapter 3, the most complete choice for thyroid treatment is desiccated thyroid (also called *glandular thyroid*, natural thyroid, natural desiccated thyroid, or NDT). Desiccated thyroid is made from the thyroid glands of pigs. It's a natural mix of all four thyroid hormones: T4, T3, T2, and T1. Thyroid medications that are synthetic—that is, made entirely from chemicals in labs—contain T4 or T3, but not T2 or T1. No one knows if T1 provides any benefits, but T2 has been found to play a role in metabolism and fat burning.

Another advantage of desiccated thyroid is that it includes significant amounts of thyroglobulin protein, which slows the dissolution of T3. This means one desiccated thyroid pill in the morning is likely to keep you going all day. In contrast, a synthetic version of T3, such as Cytomel, will lose its potency after 10 hours, so you'd typically need to take half your dosage in the morning and the other half in the late afternoon—and having to remember to do the latter without fail day after day can become burdensome.

One other positive aspect of desiccated thyroid is its low price. Pigs are raised for their meat, and until this medication was developed, pig thyroids were just thrown away, so the cost of the prime ingredient is small. Further, the market is wide open, because no one can patent the gland of an animal that's been on Earth for thousands of years. You can typically buy a one-month supply of desiccated thyroid for around $20. In fact, there's no such thing as a generic version of desiccated thyroid because the brand names are already at generic-level prices.

A potential disadvantage of desiccated thyroid is that the T4:T3 ratio in a pig thyroid is roughly 5:1, while in a human thyroid, it's roughly 13:1. In my experience, 90–95 percent of patients do fine on desiccated thyroid's higher level of T3. After all, it's the hormone that does the actual work of powering up your cells, and T4 exists merely to be converted into T3. Further, your body has ways of balancing things out, such as breaking down excess T3 into T2 and T1, and converting more of your T4 into reverse T3 instead of T3 (see Chapter 1).

If you prefer to adjust your medication's T4-to-T3 ratio, though, you can easily do so by asking your doctor to prescribe a smaller dosage of desiccated thyroid along with an appropriate amount of synthetic T4, such as Synthroid or levothyroxine. Your body makes no distinction between the T4 from desiccated thyroid and synthetic T4, so you can freely combine these medications as long as you end up with the right overall dosage.

Along the same lines, desiccated thyroid can be a bit less convenient than Synthroid in that it's not available in as many sizes. However, if you require a dosage that's not offered by your desiccated thyroid brand, you can take a mix of desiccated thyroid and Synthroid to achieve the dosage you need. (Alternatively, you can opt to cut your desiccated thyroid pills in half, as the hormones are evenly distributed throughout each pill.)

A more significant issue for desiccated thyroid is that it's not always available. While synthetic medication can be made in a lab at any time, desiccated thyroid depends on pig thyroids, and occasionally there are shortages of that porcine ingredient. When this occurs, you might have to call around to different pharmacies to find one with a supply of your medication. (If all else fails, you can briefly switch to a synthetic T4/T3 combination, such as Synthroid and Cytomel.)

Another potential downside is that you might object to the prime ingredient. For example, synthetics may be a better choice for you if your religion forbids you from consuming anything from a pig, or if you're a vegan opposed to ingesting parts of any animal, or if you simply find the idea of getting your medication from a pig to be yucky.

Perhaps the biggest disadvantage of desiccated thyroid is that many mainstream doctors will either be reluctant or will flat-out refuse to prescribe it. As just explained, there were consistency issues with desiccated thyroid before 1985, but that was decades ago. In the twenty-first century, desiccated thyroid is the most complete solution to hypothyroidism; and many doctors will accept your choice if you clearly and tactfully explain why it's your top preference.

Popular brands of desiccated thyroid include Nature-Throid and WP Thyroid from RLC Labs (RLCLabs.com). These two medications are identical, and they're marketed under different names only for historical reasons (see Chapter 3).

Another highly popular brand is Armour Thyroid from Allergan (ArmourThyroid.com). This book doesn't mention Armour Thyroid very often simply because its manufacturer stopped making it, for unknown reasons, while we were writing most of the chapters. However, Armour is now back on the market, and it's as excellent as any other natural thyroid medication.

Synthetic T4

By far the most famous thyroid medication is Synthroid, which is synthetic T4 made by Abbott (Abbott.com). Synthroid is what most doctors prescribe across the board to manage hypothyroidism. In fact, over the years, it's been one of the top 10 most-prescribed medications in America.

Synthroid is excellent at what it does—which is provide T4 in a readily available and affordable way, and in a wide range of dosages. The key question you must consider is whether T4 alone is enough for your needs.

As explained in Chapter 1, T4 is a "storage" hormone designed to circulate in your bloodstream and be constantly available to your tissues. T4 gives your body stability because the hormone is long-lasting, remaining potent for around eight days (versus just one day for T3).

When energy is called for, your body converts T4 to T3. And it's T3 that does the work of powering up your cells.

Doctors prescribe Synthroid based on two beliefs:

O Synthroid's T4 will be converted into all the T3 you need.

O T4 and T3 are all you need from your thyroid medication.

These beliefs are often validated. In my experience, roughly two-thirds of patients whose thyroids are still functioning—that is, still make a certain amount of T3 and T2—do well on Synthroid alone. (Whether they'd do subtly better on desiccated thyroid is anyone's guess....)

For roughly one third of patients, however, the T4 provided by Synthroid isn't enough. No one is sure whether it's because these patients have problems fully converting the T4 to T3, or if they simply require direct T3 in addition to direct T4 (which is what a healthy thyroid makes—again, in a roughly 1:13 ratio).

Whatever the reason, if you happen to fall into the latter category, you'll continue experiencing hypothyroid symptoms despite being on Synthroid. In this case, you should switch to either desiccated thyroid or a mix of Synthroid and Cytomel (to be described shortly).

Synthroid is the best-known T4 medication, but it's not the only one available. Others include:

O Levoxyl from Pfizer (Levoxyl.com)

O Unithroid from Amneal Pharmaceuticals (Unithroid.com)

There isn't much difference between these brand name versions of T4. The main advantages of Synthroid are that it's readily available from any pharmacy and sold in a wide range of dosages to fit any need (as detailed in Chapter 3).

Alternatively, you can buy a generic version of T4 called *levothyroxine*, which is produced by multiple manufacturers. A generic version has the same thyroid hormone as any brand name. However, because T4 is minute—much smaller than a grain of salt—it takes up less than 1 percent of a pill. The rest of the pill consists of "filler" material, and your body might absorb one type of filler material better or worse than another, which influences how effectively the T4 will enter your bloodstream.

It doesn't matter if one brand is a bit more or less effective at delivering T4 to your body, because your doctor will be tailoring your dosage based on the ultimate effect your medication is having. If you keep taking the same brand, the manufacturer makes no changes to its medication, and your thyroid's status doesn't change, you should do fine at the same dosage month after month.

The issue with generics is that your pharmacy might get pills from manufacturer X one month and manufacturer Y the next month; and because each manufacturer uses different filler material, one pill might deliver less T4 to your bloodstream than another.

If you've been taking the same generic medication month after month and notice your pharmacy has suddenly given you pills that are a different size and shape, you can perform a quick test to compare them to what you've been used to. Fill two glasses with cold water, and place one of your old pills in the first glass and one of the new pills in the second. After half an hour, check the glasses. If both pills have become equally mushy, you'll probably absorb the new medication just as well as the old one.

If you see hard chunks in the second glass, however, you'll probably absorb less T4, and over time this could lead to your hypothyroidism symptoms returning. In this case, consider switching to a pharmacy that's more consistent about supplying the same generic medication every month, or consider switching to a brand name.

That said, if you keep an eye out for your hypothyroidism symptoms returning, the risk of trying generics is low...and can save you $10–$30 a month.

Synthetic T3

If you're taking synthetic T4 such as Synthroid and want to supplement it with T3, but for some reason don't want to take desiccated thyroid, you can instead choose Cytomel from Pfizer (Pfizer.com).

Cytomel is synthetic T3. It comes in three sizes: 5, 25, and 50 micrograms. You can combine these to achieve any dosage. (For example, if you needed 35 mcg, you'd take one 25 mcg and two 5 mcg pills.)

Cytomel should be taken first thing in the morning, along with any other thyroid medication, to avoid mixing it with food. Cytomel loses its potency after about 10 hours, though, so you should ideally split your daily dosage, taking half in the morning and the other half in the late afternoon (waiting at least three hours after eating before taking the second dose).

For reasons that aren't yet fully understood, taking direct T3 such as Cytomel is especially helpful in eliminating depression. That's the case even for patients who don't appear to be hypothyroid, which is why doctors are increasingly prescribing Cytomel as a supplement to antidepressants.

Therefore, if you're exclusively on T4 and still experiencing hypothyroid symptoms, don't hesitate to ask your doctor to add Cytomel to your prescription. Even doctors who are hardcore Synthroid advocates will generally be willing to supplement it with Cytomel.

Alternatively, you can purchase a generic version named *liothyronine*, which is up to three times less expensive. In most cases, the generic will be just as effective as the brand name version. However, as discussed in the previous section, beware of your pharmacy using generics from different manufacturers from month to month, which can create variable results.

On the other side of the expense spectrum, you can purchase a time-released version of synthetic T3 from a *liothyronine* compounding pharmacy. This spares you from having to take the medication more than once a day. However, there are serious risks involved (see Chapter 3).

Another downside to compounding pharmacies is that most of them aren't equipped to perform post-production analysis. That's significant, because brand name manufacturers end up rejecting as much as 20 percent of their thyroid pills due to the medication not passing quality control standards. That means as much as one in five thyroid pills from a compounding pharmacy might have too little or too much thyroid hormone.

Combining T4 and T3

Recognizing that many people do better on a combination of T4 and T3 medication than on T4 alone, and that there was an audience for a Kosher- and vegan-friendly alternative to desiccated thyroid, for decades Forest Labs produced a synthetic T4/T3 medication named Thyrolar. However, the manufacturer missed opportunities to make this product stand out from the crowd. For example, it could've made Thyrolar's T4:T3 mix like the 13:1 ratio of a human thyroid. Instead, it chose a ratio of 4:1, mimicking the inhumanly high level of T3 that's arguably the least appealing aspect of desiccated thyroid. Thyrolar was discontinued in 2018.

That said, Synthroid and Cytomel—as well as their generic versions—are still readily available, and you can combine them in any T4 to T3 ratio that suits your needs.

Arguably, an ideal synthetic thyroid medication would mix T4 and T3 in a 13:1 ratio, include small amounts of T2 and T1, and always be available for purchase. But no such product currently exists; and considering the cost for a new drug seeking FDA approval can easily exceed $500 million, such a product is unlikely to appear anytime soon.

Meanwhile, the medication closest to this ideal is a mix of desiccated thyroid and synthetic T4.

For example, a 55-year-old patient of mine named Marti had been stable for several years on a 90 milligram (mg) dose of Nature-Throid. While going through a divorce, Marti came to see me about persistent anxiety. Her anxiousness wasn't unusual under the circumstances, so we mostly focused on lifestyle changes to reduce stress. For safety's sake, though, I took some of Marti's blood for testing.

The results showed Marti's cortisol levels had gone up, which is something that can happen in response to acute stress. Initially, Cortisol can speed the conversion of T4 into T3 (though over time it'll block T3 from accessing cells, leading to hypothyroidism—see Chapter 14). Because Marti was getting too much T3, but I didn't want to lower her T4, I adjusted her medication from 90 mg of Nature-Throid to a mix of 30 mg of Nature-Throid and 88 micrograms (mcg) of levothyroxine (generic T4). After a couple of months, Marti's anxiety faded away.

You should never settle for less than optimal treatment. If your symptoms continue while on one type of medication, insist that your doctor let you try something else.

And if your symptoms go away but then recur, or you experience new symptoms, don't hesitate to return to your doctor for retesting.

With all the options available for treating hypothyroidism, you should be able to lead a life just as rich and symptom-free as that of anyone with a perfectly healthy thyroid.

Beyond Prescription Medication

Thyroid medication is the primary remedy for hypothyroidism, but it's not the only one.

Chapter 18, "Reversing Thyroid Disease Through Diet," explains how to enhance your treatment by adopting a vegan or vegan-like diet for at least 3–6 months. While the process takes work and perseverance, it might slow or stop the damage being done to your thyroid, help your thyroid heal, and eventually mitigate or eliminate your need for medication.

And just in case your thyroid issue is at least partially being caused by an infection, consider trying over-the-counter antiviral/antibacterial supplements to see if they make you feel better. Popular supplements include vitamin C (1,000–2,000 mg, taken with food to avoid upsetting your stomach), cat's claw, L-lysine, lemon balm, and goldenseal (taken at the dosages recommended on their respective labels).

Then again, you might be low on selenium, which is a key chemical your body uses to convert T4 to T3 (see Chapter 1). If you aren't sure whether you have enough selenium, you can check via a *red blood cell element test*. This is a highly informative blood test that measures your 3-month average levels of essential chemicals boron, chromium, calcium, copper, iron, magnesium, manganese, molybdenum, phosphorus, potassium, selenium, vanadium, and zinc. It also detects the presence of the toxins arsenic, cadmium, lead, mercury, and thallium. (For more on toxins, see Chapters 18 and 20.) The test costs around $250. If it turns up a selenium shortage, you can easily solve it by eating one Brazil nut daily.

Then again, you can opt to skip the test and simply commit to eating the Brazil nut, just in case. (Don't eat more than one a day regularly, though, or you could end up overdosing.)

One other approach that requires zero medicine is a yoga posture called the *shoulder stand*. If you're fit to do yoga, you can perform this by lying flat on your back, letting your body rest on your shoulders and the back of your neck, and raising your legs together until they're pointing straight up. It's a little like doing a headstand, but instead of the top of your head, you're using the back of your neck, with your chin pressed hard against your chest. This places substantial compression on your thyroid and can increase the blood supply to it.

If any of these remedies help you, then you might end up with a thyroid that's either less dependent on medication or doesn't need medication at all.

In the meantime, though, you should be on prescription meds to help protect your thyroid, feel good, and live a normal life; and taking the right dosage is critical. The next chapter will guide you in selecting your level of thyroid medication, as well as how to seamlessly switch from one brand to another.

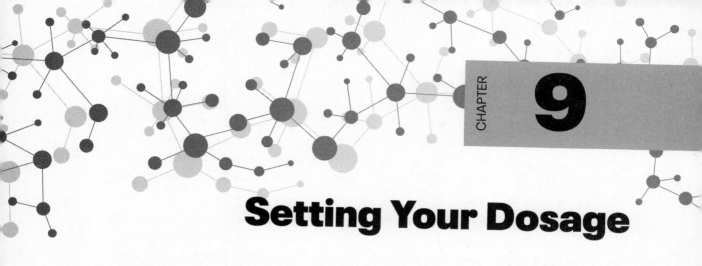

Setting Your Dosage

Chapter 8 helped you choose your thyroid medication. Your final step to health is deciding precisely how much medication you need. If you don't take enough medication, you'll continue having hypothyroidism symptoms. But if you take too much medication, you'll become hyperthyroid, which is a much more dangerous illness (see Chapter 10).

This chapter explains what you need to know to avoid undesirable extremes and arrive at the dosage that's perfect for you.

Finding Your Perfect Dosage

Discovering precisely the right amount of thyroid medication you need is a process of educated guesswork and trial and error, using your symptoms and blood tests as ways of continually checking on whether a choice is closer to or further from your optimal dosage.

The first factor to consider is your weight. A very rough rule of thumb is that your body needs one microgram (mcg) of T4, or its equivalent, per pound (up to 300 pounds). That means an adult weighing 200 pounds will need roughly 175–225 mcg of total thyroid hormones, while an adult weighing 150 pounds will need roughly 125–175 mcg.

The other key factor is how much help your thyroid needs. For example, if you're in the early stages of thyroid disease, you might require just a little bit of medication to make up for your thyroid's moderate underactivity. However, your doctor might have to gradually increase your dosage over time if your thyroid grows progressively worse.

Then again, if your thyroid has entirely stopped working, or has been surgically removed, your medication will need to take the place of *all* the hormones a thyroid normally supplies. The good news is there isn't much of a practical difference between being on lower or higher dose pills—they typically cost the same, are around the same size, and have the same rules. (Take them first thing in the morning with nothing but water.)

There's even a distinct advantage to fully replacing a shut down or missing thyroid with medication, which is that once you determine the dosage that's right for you, it's unlikely to change. This means unless you notice symptoms returning—or new symptoms—you won't need to have your thyroid hormone levels checked more than once a year.

You and your doctor can determine to what extent your thyroid needs help via two diagnostic tools: your thyroid blood tests (see Chapter 7) and your symptoms (see Chapter 6).

After studying the results of your initial blood tests, your doctor will prescribe her best guess for an appropriate dosage. She'll err on the low side because there's no danger to your being slightly hypothyroid, while there *are* serious hazards associated with long-term hyperthyroidism, including heart damage and bone loss. For this reason, your doctor will ask you to be alert for hyperthyroidism symptoms, such as a rapidly beating heart, acute anxiety, or feeling like you drank a pot of coffee when you didn't.

It can take up to three months for your medication to clearly show up as a new TSH level in your bloodstream. However, in half that time your new free T4 and free T3 levels will have stabilized, and your TSH level might at least have started shifting; so to ensure you aren't seriously over or under your therapeutic level, your doctor will typically ask you to come back in around six weeks.

Shortly before your second visit, pay attention to your body while skimming through Chapter 2. If you notice any symptoms that you reasonably believe might be caused by either hypothyroidism or hyperthyroidism, jot them down, and be prepared to describe them when your doctor asks how you feel. If your doctor is a good one, she'll take your symptoms into account along with her physical examination and the results of your second round of blood tests. She'll then use all this information to fine-tune your dosage.

It's common to need a bit less medication but feel as though you need a bit more, and vice versa. But if you changed your dosage on your own, you'd be making a small problem into a bigger one. Instead, simply rely on your feeling that *something* is wrong, and see your doctor for another round of blood tests. The combination of symptoms, a brief physical exam, and lab results will provide a clear view of the current state of your hypothyroidism.

If the change to your dosage is smaller than what you expected, be aware that these corrections are akin to steering a big ship. If you turn a ship's wheel too drastically, you'll soon end up off course. Similarly, when your lab numbers are close to where they should be, doctors prefer gentle and gradual modifications that yield significant results over a month or two.

After your second visit, your doctor will probably ask to see you again in three months, this time allowing for your TSH level to fully reflect your latest dosage change.

If your dosage requires only minor adjustments after your third visit, your doctor will probably ask to see you again in 6–12 months.

No matter when your next visit is scheduled, you should never hesitate to make an earlier appointment if you notice symptoms returning or getting worse, or new symptoms appearing. Aside from any risks involved, there's no good reason for you to spend weeks feeling awful when a simple modification of your dosage can restore your good health.

Be Goldilocks

Most doctors beware extremes in either direction, and you should too—even when they come from your own physician. For example, if a man weighs 180 pounds and his thyroid has shut down, and he's prescribed 50 mcg of Synthroid, that's way too low for even a conservative initial dosage. Similarly, if you're feeling awful for over three months on an exceptionally low dosage and your doctor tells you to be patient, you should find another doctor.

As another example, if your practitioner tells you to take more than three grains of Nature-Throid—the equivalent of 300 mcg of Synthroid—that's flat-out dangerous (aside from rare circumstances, such as if you weigh well over 300 pounds). If you went along with this dosage recommendation, it would plunge you into hyperthyroidism and put you at risk of a heart attack.

Some alternative medicine practitioners rely solely on symptoms and basal temperature (see Chapter 3), and might prescribe daily doses of four grains, five grains, six grains, and more of desiccated thyroid.

Overdosing makes many people feel awful, but some patients become accustomed to the overstimulation. Periodically, I'll see a patient who's on more than three grains of medication who tells me he feels great. I'll respond, "You might feel great on cocaine, too. That doesn't mean it's good for you." A stimulant is making your body become more active than is normal, and that's not sustainable. At some point, a crash is inevitable.

My first step with such a patient is to taper him off the overdosing as quickly as possible without shocking his system. Sometimes patients come to me too late, however. In as little as six months, serious damage can be done to the heart and bones; plus it's not unusual for such a patient to enter a permanent state of hyperthyroidism, such as Graves' disease.

Don't let this happen to you. Like Goldilocks, steer clear of too little and too much, and stay focused on finding the dosage that's just right for your body's needs.

Mixing and Switching Thyroid Medications

As Chapter 8 explained, you have a variety of thyroid medications to choose from, and you can mix these thyroid medications however you like to achieve the type of dosage you desire. That's because your body makes no distinctions between synthetic and natural hormones, or between brand name and generic hormones.

Along the same lines, you can freely switch from one medication to another, as long as you choose the equivalent dosage. If you encounter any transition issues, they'll typically be because over 99 percent of any thyroid hormone pill consists of inactive filler material, and you might find that some fillers make it easier for your body to absorb the active hormones in pills than others (see Chapter 3).

You can see which dosage of thyroid medication is equivalent to the dosage of another medication using the following table:

Thyroid Medication Conversion Guide

T4: Synthroid/ Levothyroxine	T3: Cytomel/ Liothyronine	WP Thyroid/ Nature-Throid	Armour
25 mcg	6.25 mcg	16.25 mg ¼ grain	15 mg ¼ grain
50 mcg	12.5 mcg	32.5 mg ½ grain	30 mg ½ grain
100 mcg	25 mcg	65 mg 1 grain	60 mg 1 grain
200 mcg	50 mcg	130 mg 2 grains	120 mg 2 grains
300 mcg	75 mcg	195 mg 3 grains	180 mg 3 grains

Please note the following details about the Conversion Guide:

O Mcg = micrograms; mg = milligrams (1 mg = 1,000 mcg); grain = 65 mg for Nature-Throid/WP Thyroid and 60 mg for Armour Thyroid.

O Nature-Throid and WP Thyroid are identical medications (see Chapter 3).

O There's a slight dosage difference between Nature-Throid/WP Thyroid (1 grain = 65 mg) and Armour Thyroid (1 grain = 60 mg).

O All medications are available as pills in the precise dosages listed *except* for Cytomel (and its generic equivalent liothyronine), which is sold only in 5 mcg, 25 mcg, and 50 mcg dosages. You can create other dosages by cutting and/or combining Cytomel pills.

O T3 is roughly four times as potent as T4—for example, 25 mcg of Cytomel = 100 mcg of Synthroid.

You should be aware that 2 + 2 = 5 when it comes to desiccated thyroid. For example, a 65 mg (1 grain) pill of Nature-Throid contains 38 mcg of T4 and 9 mcg of T3. Given that T3 is about four times as potent as T4, that works out to 74 mcg (38 mcg + 36 mcg) of T4. However, the Conversion Guide shows that a 65 mg pill of

Nature-Throid is equivalent to a 100 mcg pill of T4. This fact comes from doctors who have decades of experience with patients switching between thyroid medications, and you'll find the same information in virtually any other conversion guide (for example, the RLC Labs guide at GetRealThyroid.com/conversion-guide.html).

You might reasonably ask where the extra 26 mcg is coming from. The truth is no one really knows. However, experts suspect that the T2 and T1 in desiccated thyroid account for its "hidden" extra power.

It's important to be aware of this discrepancy between desiccated thyroid's stated active ingredients and its actual potency. If your doctor isn't experienced with desiccated thyroid, he might look at only the active ingredients and prescribe too much for you. You should therefore always refer to the Conversion Guide when switching between medications...and, if necessary, bring it to your doctor's attention.

Real Patient Dosage Stories

It can be easier to understand the process of selecting the right dosage within the context of people's lives. The following are true stories of patients who required medication for their hypothyroidism. They were all restored to full health once they stabilized on the right dosage.

Total Thyroid Hormone Replacement

Dan had a perfectly functioning thyroid. Unfortunately, it developed cancer. To eradicate the disease, it was necessary to surgically remove the thyroid.

I normally ease a patient onto medication gradually. This wasn't appropriate in Dan's case, however, because we needed to entirely replace the hormones previously produced by his otherwise healthy thyroid.

Dan weighed 200 pounds, so my initial guess was that he needed the equivalent of 200 mcg of T4 daily. The ways Dan could've received this dosage include:

○ **Synthetic T4:** 200 mcg Synthroid pill, or 200 mcg levothyroxine (generic T4) pill

○ **Synthetic T4 and T3 mix:** 100 mcg Synthroid pill and 25 mcg Cytomel pill, or 100 mcg levothyroxine (generic T4) pill and 25 mcg liothyronine (generic T3) pill

○ **Natural T4, T3, T2, and T1:** Desiccated thyroid via a 130 mg (2 grain) Nature-Throid or WP Thyroid pill, or a 120 mg (2 grain) Armour Thyroid pill

Because the only way for Dan to get both a normal amount of T2 and a time-released version of T3 was via desiccated thyroid, I suggested a 130 mg (2 grain) pill of Nature-Throid daily. Dan agreed. Subsequent months of testing—and lack of symptoms—showed that this was just the right medication and dosage for him.

Underdose for Depression

Lori's problem was depression. She'd tried four major antidepressants, but none of them worked for her. When Lori came to me for help, she mentioned that she'd been taking 75 mcg of Synthroid for the past five years. That's a small amount for most adults, so I immediately suspected underdosing as the source of Lori's ills.

Blood tests confirmed this; Lori's TSH was high and her hormone levels were below normal. I raised her prescription to 100 mcg of Synthroid and asked Lori to come in for another round of testing in three months. I also told her to come in right away if she noticed any signs of hyperthyroidism, such as her heart rate increasing.

Three months later, Lori's depression had largely lifted. However, she was now complaining of fatigue. When I questioned her, it turned out that once Lori had started feeling better, she'd begun training for a marathon—on top of taking a full load of courses for a master's degree! When the lab results came in, they showed Lori's TSH and thyroid hormone levels were now perfect. I explained to Lori that it was simply her newfound enthusiasm for life that was wearing her out. Once Lori adjusted to being healthy again, she was fine on the 100 mcg dosage.

Overdose for Fatigue

Josie was feeling severely fatigued. She first saw a doctor who followed the principles of Broda Barnes (see Chapter 3). Using only the basal temperature test, he diagnosed her as hypothyroid and prescribed a 120 mg (2 grain) pill of Armour Thyroid. When these had no effect, he progressively raised her dosage, telling Josie that her symptoms would be resolved once she had enough thyroid hormones.

When Josie was up to 240 mg (4 grains) of Armour Thyroid daily, her heart was pounding in her chest and she was periodically fainting. At that point she came to see me for a second opinion.

I first told Josie that we needed to immediately taper her off the extreme overdose she'd been prescribed. I added that because she was feeling just as much fatigue as before, there was a good chance her problem was never caused by her thyroid at all.

I took Josie's blood and ordered a series of tests. A few days later, the results showed Josie was in the late stages of Addison's disease (see Chapter 14).

I helped wean Josie completely off her thyroid medication and placed her on medication that directly addressed her adrenal disease. After six months, Josie was feeling enormously better.

A Dog's Tale

Margie was doing fine on her thyroid medication, so I was surprised to get a panicked call from her toward the end of a warm summer day. All my nurse told me was that there'd been an overdose.

"Hello, Margie," I said. "Are you okay?"

"I'm fine," she said. "But I keep my Armour pills by the bed, and my dog knocked the bottle over while I was away at work and ate them all. There was a two-week supply in there! I'm afraid he's going to die!"

I shook my head. "It's probably the mild pig smell that attracted him. This happens from time to time."

"He's running around chasing his tail! Should I rush him to the emergency room?"

"It would do no harm to have him checked by your vet," I said, "but he'll probably be fine. Dogs use a lot more thyroid hormone per pound than people. The most important thing you can do is put the pills where he can't get at them in the future."

"Like where?" Margie asked.

"You can store them in the freezer," I said. "Not only will it prevent your dog from accessing the pills, it'll end their mild odor, so he won't even be interested in them when you take them out in the morning. It's probably the warm summer day—which caused some of the pills' molecules to drift into the air—that made him go after them in the first place."

If you have children at home, similar advice applies—always keep your thyroid medication in a safe place where no one can reach them but you. All the reasons for you to avoid an overdose—risk of heart damage, your thyroid shutting down, etc.—go double for young ones.

Staying on Your Medication

After meeting all the challenges involved with hypothyroidism—identifying the disease, getting the right tests done, interpreting the lab results correctly, choosing the appropriate medication, and determining the perfect dosage—you'd think that patients would take their pills without fail every morning.

Oddly enough, though, some don't. Once their symptoms have gone away, their pills run out, and nothing terrible immediately happens, a certain number of patients fail to renew their medication because they feel like they've been "cured."

In fact, hypothyroidism is usually a long-term disease if a patient relies on medication alone (see Chapter 18). Within anywhere from a week to a couple of months of no treatment, its symptoms will return. This can happen so slowly and subtly that it's not immediately obvious. Making matters worse is that one of the symptoms is often a slowing of mental faculties that affects judgment. As a result, someone can be suffering for quite a while before realizing what's happening.

You should therefore virtually never go off your medication unless your doctor tells you it's okay to do so. The only exception is if you're experiencing symptoms of hyperthyroidism; and in this case, you should call your doctor immediately to get advice and make an appointment.

As long as you stay on your medication, pay close attention to your body for hypothyroidism symptoms, and see your doctor for a physical exam and blood tests at least once a year, you should be able to live as rich and healthy a life as anyone with a perfectly functioning thyroid.

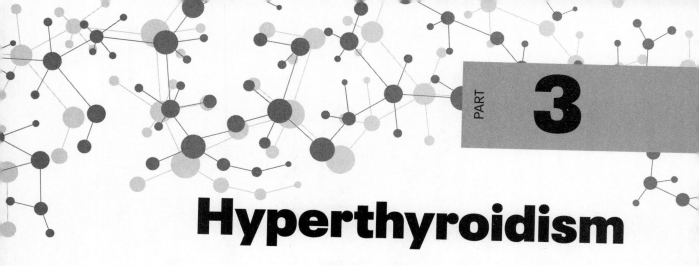

Hyperthyroidism

In this part we focus on hyperthyroidism, which can make you feel as if you're perpetually drinking a big pot of black coffee.

Chapter 10 describes typical symptoms—racing heart, anxiety, tremors—and the various types of hyperthyroidism.

Chapter 11 explains how to diagnose and test for hyperthyroidism.

And Chapter 12 covers how to treat hyperthyroidism.

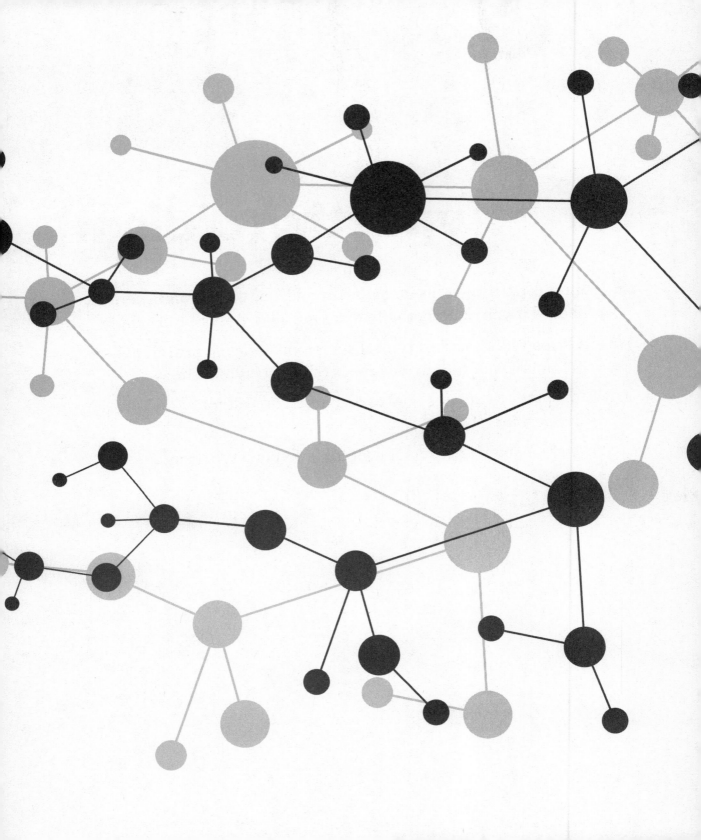

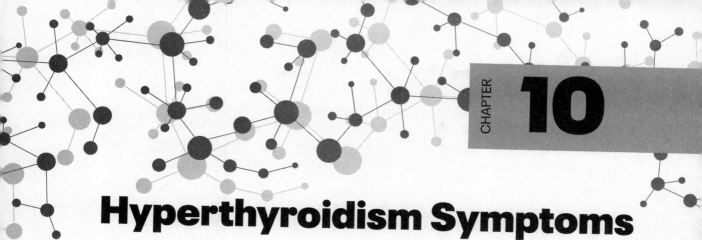

Hyperthyroidism Symptoms

If your heart is racing, you're feeling anxious, you're losing weight for no apparent reason, or you're experiencing any of dozens of other symptoms, you might be *hyperthyroid*.

More than 90,000 Americans every year are diagnosed with hyperthyroidism, and millions of people suffer from it worldwide. It strikes over five times as many women as men, and the odds of becoming hyperthyroid increase with age.

In addition to those genetically disposed to the disease, hyperthyroidism is an ever-present danger for the tens of millions of people being treated for hypothyroidism. That's because your body reacts the same whether you have an overactive thyroid or consume too much thyroid medication.

This is the first of three chapters providing you with the knowledge you need to meet the various challenges posed by hyperthyroidism. Once you've read these chapters, you'll know whether you should see a doctor, and how to make sure you receive the best testing, diagnosis, and treatment.

Hyperthyroidism Symptoms Checklist

As explained in Chapter 1, your thyroid regulates the energy level of every cell in your body through the production of its hormones. Hyperthyroidism occurs when the levels of those hormones are above normal. In fact, the first part of this disease's name, *hyper*, is Greek for *over* (just as *hyper*active refers to being overly active).

The excess hormones increase the activity of cells throughout your body, which can be so overstimulating that you might feel as if you're perpetually drinking a big pot of black coffee.

Because thyroid hormones affect every cell, in theory, an overactive thyroid can result in any of hundreds of symptoms. In general, though, certain symptoms are more likely to occur than others. These frequent clues to hyperthyroidism appear in the checklist that follows.

Take a few minutes to go over the list and check off any symptom that applies to you. If you aren't sure whether you have a symptom, find the description of it in Chapter 2, and also see if it's covered in the patient stories that follow. Use that additional information to make your decision.

Hyperthyroidism Symptoms Checklist

- Severe anxiety and panic attacks
- Irritability
- Shakiness, including hand tremors
- Heart pounding more than 90 beats per minute while at rest
- A racing mind that makes it difficult to focus
- Insomnia
- Losing weight for no apparent reason (or gaining weight due to an abrupt increase in appetite)
- Feeling overheated

- Oversweating (especially in the head, hands, and feet)
- Tingling in the hands and feet
- Frequent bowel movements and/or a loose stool
- Menstrual problems
- A sex drive that's in overdrive
- Weak muscles
- Thinning hair
- Thyroid growths (goiters)
- Eyes sensitive to light
- A dry, gritty feeling in the eyes
- Enlarged, protruding eyes (creating a "bug-eyed" look)

If you have six or more of these common symptoms, there's a strong chance you're hyperthyroid. Get your thyroid checked out—typically via blood tests for TSH, free T4, free T3, and thyroid antibodies—as soon as possible.

If you have two to five of these symptoms, that's still reason enough to get your thyroid tested. Either the results will be positive, putting you on the path to treatment, or they'll be negative, which will inform your doctor to explore another source for the problems.

But even if you have only one of these symptoms and your doctor isn't providing a satisfying explanation for its cause, you should seriously consider getting tested. That's especially true if you're a woman, as your risk is five times greater than a man of being struck by hyperthyroidism.

The checklist is by no means comprehensive; you can experience other symptoms. However, the odds are that along with the unlisted symptoms, you'll have at least a few of the ones on the checklist—and these are all the clues you need to go get tested.

If you're successfully treated, you'll soon experience improvement regarding *all* your hyperthyroidism symptoms.

Some of the symptoms on the checklist apply to both hyperthyroidism and hypothyroidism—for example, insomnia, weak muscles, thinning hair, goiters, menstrual problems, and gaining weight. In each case, the problem stems from different causes but has the same result. Fortunately, all you need to do is see a doctor who'll test your blood for thyroid disease. The lab results will reveal your condition.

Hyperthyroidism Dangers

Some people enjoy being hyperthyroid at first. During its initial, milder stages you can become unusually productive, especially at low-level tasks like cleaning out the garage. But at a certain point hyperthyroidism may become not only unpleasant, but horrific.

For example, one of my patients was a photojournalist who risked his life covering wars and taking pictures of soldiers during combat. He told me the anxiety he experienced was so gut-wrenching that he'd felt safer and more comfortable being shot at on battlefields than he did sitting at home with his family during hyperthyroid-induced panic attacks.

As another example, early on in my career I took thyroid medication I didn't need to understand what my hyperthyroid patients were going through. It was one of the worst experiences of my life. Perhaps it made me a better doctor, but I wouldn't recommend anyone willingly going through such an ordeal.

In addition to the overt symptoms, hyperthyroidism can cause bone loss (osteoporosis), cardiovascular damage that can lead to a heart attack, and pressure on ocular nerves that can eventually lead to blindness.

In fact, one of the few advantages of hyperthyroidism is that it's not subtle. Especially in its later stages, its symptoms are so severe that most doctors can quickly spot them and identify their causes.

Otherwise, as awful as hypothyroidism is, hyperthyroidism is worse. In fact, among the prime cures for hyperthyroidism is turning you hypothyroid instead—typically via drugs, surgery, or radiation that reduces your thyroid's functionality. At that point, your condition can be managed via hypothyroid medication.

Graves' Disease

Roughly 80 percent of hyperthyroidism results from *Graves' disease,* a condition in which the thyroid undergoes attacks that cause it to overproduce its hormones.

This grim-sounding illness doesn't derive its name from its outcome—it's highly treatable—but from an Irish doctor named Robert James Graves who was the first to write about it in detail in 1835.

Graves' disease strikes women about seven times as often as men. It most commonly occurs during early adolescence and ages 30–50, but it can happen at any age.

Graves' is considered to be an *autoimmune* disease. The medical community believes it occurs when your immune system—which normally protects you by attacking foreign invaders such as viruses and bacteria—mistakes your thyroid as a danger and starts attacking it, too.

The primary suspected trigger for Graves' disease is an excess of iodine, the key chemical your thyroid uses to make its hormones. Your thyroid is designed to sift through your blood, and suck in and store even the tiniest amounts of iodine it finds. This ability is normally wonderful, because it means you need to consume only a little bit of iodine daily to have enough T3 and T4.

If you have a genetic disposition for Graves', however, your thyroid's sensitivity to iodine may cause your immune system to identify even a mild overdose as toxic...and send antibodies to attack.

As with Hashimoto's disease (see Chapter 5), this might involve *thyroid peroxidase* antibodies and *thyroglobulin* antibodies. But the primary cause of Graves' is *thyroid stimulating immunoglobulin* antibodies, or *TSI*. TSI is unique because while it's attacking your thyroid's cells, it's stimulating them into producing more hormones.

TSI has essentially the same effect as the *thyroid stimulating hormone*, or *TSH*, secreted by your pituitary gland (see Chapter 1). However, while TSH production is linked to the amount of T3 and T4 in your bloodstream and is designed to maintain balanced thyroid hormone levels, TSI is produced with no regard to your body's thyroid levels, and with no limits. In other words, TSI is like a rogue, insane version of your pituitary gland; and it makes your thyroid produce much more T3 and T4 than your body needs.

Graves' disease has a lot in common with Hashimoto's disease—they're both autoimmune thyroid conditions, and they're both responsible for most thyroid disease. The key difference is that the antibodies that cause Hashimoto's attack the inner proteins of the thyroid, which breaks down its cells. In contrast, Graves' is caused by TSI antibodies that attack the thyroid's receptors for TSH—and in the process, continually stimulates them. Even after your pituitary gland shuts down in response to your body having too much T3 and T4, the stimulation from the TSI ensures your thyroid will continue to overproduce hormones and keep you hyperthyroid.

The results include all the symptoms of hyperthyroidism previously described—elevated heart rate, panic attacks, tremors, etc. In addition, the extra activity frequently leads to one or more *goiters,* which are enlargements of your thyroid, and to eye problems.

If left untreated, Graves' will become progressively more severe. Fortunately, there are a variety of treatment options for this disease (see Chapters 12 and 18).

Goitrous Hyperthyroidism

A goiter is a non-cancerous swelling on your thyroid. Your thyroid can grow one or multiple goiters. This condition isn't really a disease; it's a side effect of diseases such as Graves'.

If you're hyperthyroid, you'll typically develop goiters when TSI antibodies relentlessly stimulate your thyroid to overproduce. Because your thyroid can't make enough hormones to meet the antibodies' demands at its current size, it grows more cells. This is an effective response when you're healthy because producing additional T3 and T4 until your bloodstream has enough will end your body's requests for these hormones. However, no amount of overproduction will satisfy the limitless demands of the TSI antibodies, which means TSI will make your thyroid keep growing and growing.

If your hyperthyroidism is successfully treated in its early stages with medication, any existing goiters will stop getting bigger, and might even fade away over time. That's because once the TSI stimulation ends, your thyroid will stop replacing dying goiter cells with fresh ones, resulting in natural shrinkage. Alternatively, if your treatment involves surgery or radiation, any goiters can be removed or destroyed as part of the procedure.

Hyperthyroid Eye Disease

If you're hyperthyroid, you're almost certain to have "lid lag." Your doctor can spot this by having you follow her finger as she moves it up and down. If the white part of your eye can be seen above your iris as you look down, it's a strong indication you're hyperthyroid.

If you have Graves' disease, there's also a roughly 30 percent chance that you'll develop more severe eye problems. For example, you can become sensitive to light. You may feel a painful dryness or grittiness in your eyes. Or you may experience double vision (called *diplopia*).

As the disease progresses, your eyelids might retract, and your eyes enlarge and protrude, creating a "bug-eyed" look. If left untreated, this is a serious condition that can put pressure on your optic nerves and eventually lead to blindness. If treatment occurs soon enough, distended eyeballs will return to normal on their own after the disease is under control. Past a certain point of growth, though, surgery might be required.

If your Graves' eye disease has been brought under control, stay alert for any signs of its return. Graves' eye disease can come back, and grow worse, even when all your other hyperthyroidism symptoms are being well managed.

Plummer's Disease

Plummer's disease is the second most common cause of hyperthyroidism. It occurs most often in women, and after age 50. Named after acclaimed American endocrinologist Henry Stanley Plummer (who co-founded the Mayo Clinic), Plummer's disease is caused by one or more non-cancerous thyroid growths, or *nodules*, that produce hormones independently—that is, without waiting to be stimulated by TSH. These nodules are referred to as "toxic" because they churn out hormones at such high levels that they'll make you hyperthyroid.

A single toxic nodule is called *Plummer's adenoma* (adenoma is another name for a non-cancerous growth). Plummer's disease can also take the form of a *toxic multinodular goiter*, in which a number of nodules spring up on a goiter.

Plummer's disease can be triggered by an abrupt large amount of iodine. This is covered in the next section.

Iodine-Induced Hyperthyroidism

Taking in an excessive amount of iodine can put you at risk of becoming hyperthyroid. This most commonly happens if you already have thyroid nodules. The iodine overload can transform existing harmless nodules into a "toxic" state in which they produce hormones independently. If the excess iodine is withdrawn, this can be a temporary condition. If you're over 50, though, just one incident can be the trigger for a permanent condition such as Plummer's disease.

For example, a 62-year-old patient named Ricardo came to see me when he was having increasingly frequent bowel movements and very loose stools for no apparent reason. When I checked his pulse, Ricardo's resting heart rate was 100.

Considering Ricardo's age and hyperthyroid symptoms, I asked him if he'd recently had any imaging tests for which he'd been given an injection. He told me that he'd had a CT scan a few months ago that used iodine to help create a clear contrast.

I took Ricardo's blood, ordered hyperthyroidism testing, and prescribed an ultrasound for his neck. I wasn't surprised when the lab results showed low TSH and high T4 levels. Thyroid antibodies were negative, ruling out Graves' disease. And a single nodule actively producing hormones was visible via the ultrasound, which confirmed my suspicion of Plummer's disease.

Within the first month of treatment, Ricardo's heart rate settled, and his bowel movements returned to normal.

Painful Subacute Thyroiditis

If your thyroid feels inflamed, you might have *painful subacute thyroiditis.* This typically occurs following a respiratory infection—for example, after you've had the mumps, the flu, or some other virus. If your body's attacks on the virus create high inflammation, this can, in turn, spawn antibodies that end up attacking your thyroid.

As your thyroid cells are destroyed, the hormones they stored are abruptly released into your bloodstream, making you hyperthyroid. This condition tends to be temporary. However, you should be treated for its symptoms until it goes away on its own.

More information about this disease—as well as other forms of thyroiditis that include stages of hyperthyroidism—appears in Chapter 15.

Hashitoxicosis

Hashitoxicosis stems from Hashimoto's disease, which is an autoimmune disease that attacks your thyroid cells (see Chapter 5). As the cells are destroyed, the hormones they stored are abruptly released into your bloodstream, making you hyperthyroid.

However, this is a temporary state. With treatment, you might be able to end the attacks. Otherwise, as Hashimoto's continues its assault over months, your thyroid will eventually become so damaged that it lapses into a permanent stage of hypothyroidism.

Thyrotoxicosis Factitia

Thyrotoxicosis factitia is a condition in which hyperthyroidism occurs as a result of artificial rather than natural causes. The most typical cause is an overdose of thyroid medication. Taking in too much T4 and/or T3 via pills has the same effect on your body as an overactive thyroid that makes too much of its hormones.

A patient can intentionally overdose in a misguided attempt to lose weight, or to overwhelmingly combat some other hypothyroid symptom. It's also possible to overdose by simply staying on your thyroid medication without sufficiently frequent testing. Sometimes, your thyroid will grow healthier with treatment and begin producing higher levels of hormones, which is a good thing; but unless your doctor detects this and decreases your dosage accordingly, you'll end up taking more medication than you need.

The simple solution to these situations is to stop taking the excess hormones. The hyperthyroidism symptoms will then usually go away on their own. If the overdosing goes on for months, though, there's a risk of triggering permanent hyperthyroidism.

In rare cases, it's also possible to consume excess thyroid hormones from meat. There have been at least two outbreaks in which the thyroid tissue in neck muscles were accidentally ground up along with other cow parts for burger patties. These resulted in "hamburger hyperthyroidism" for entire communities.

TSH-Secreting Pituitary Adenoma

Less than 1 percent of hyperthyroidism cases are caused by a condition called *TSH-secreting pituitary adenoma.* As explained in Chapter 1, your thyroid's activities are regulated by your pituitary gland. When your body is running low on energy, your pituitary gland secretes TSH to tell your thyroid to get to work and make more hormones.

This is a great system when everything is working normally. However, just as your thyroid can grow a toxic nodule, the pituitary gland can develop a non-cancerous growth (an adenoma) that turns rogue and independently produces TSH. In contrast to your pituitary generating TSH based on your body's needs, the adenoma arbitrarily makes excessive amounts of TSH.

All TSH looks alike to your thyroid, so it'll obey the orders of the adenoma just as fully as the ones from your pituitary gland. Even though your thyroid is healthy, you'll end up with way too much T3 and T4, and become hyperthyroid.

You might also experience other things going wrong. For example, in addition to thyroid hormones, your pituitary gland is responsible for regulating the production of prolactin. Therefore—even if you're a man—you might abruptly start lactating, which normally occurs only in women after childbirth.

The presence of a pituitary adenoma can be picked up by blood tests that show both high TSH and high levels of thyroid hormones. Because TSH and T4/T3 normally have an inverse relationship—when one is high, the other is low, and vice versa—all levels being high indicates an out-of-control pituitary gland whose TSH production is no longer fully connected to your body's needs. The condition can then be confirmed by an MRI of your pituitary gland, which will show an active adenoma growing on it.

If the adenoma is small—under 14 millimeters—it can often be shrunk down until it's harmless via such medications as bromocriptine and cabergoline.

Otherwise, you'll require surgery on your pituitary gland to remove the adenoma. This is especially important because in addition to making you hyperthyroid, continued growth of the adenoma threatens to put pressure on and damage your nearby optic nerves.

Struma Ovarii

In very rare cases—well under 1 percent—a woman can develop an ovarian tumor with thyroid tissue called *struma*. Thyroid cells don't belong in the ovaries, but sometimes cells grow in inappropriate places. If the struma is distinct enough to not respond to TSH but similar enough to your thyroid to produce hormones, the excess T3 and T4 will make you hyperthyroid. This condition is treated by surgical removal of the struma.

If at this point you suspect that you're hyperthyroid, it's very important that you get tested and diagnosed. The next chapter covers this process.

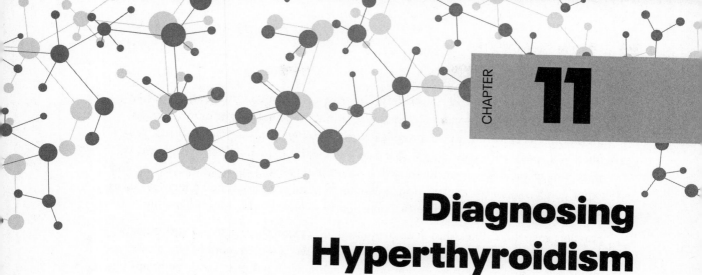

11

Diagnosing Hyperthyroidism

If you're experiencing one or more of the symptoms described in Chapter 10 and believe the cause might be hyperthyroidism, you shouldn't hesitate to see a doctor and get tested.

The initial phase of this process is straightforward—your doctor takes some of your blood, then sends it to a lab with instructions on which tests to run. What makes things a bit complicated is that many doctors fail to ask for the right combination of tests. In addition, some doctors fail to sufficiently consider all possible causes.

This chapter guides you through the hyperthyroidism diagnostic process. It first discusses conditions that resemble hyperthyroidism and might account for your symptoms. It then details the best testing and analysis methods for determining whether you're hyperthyroid.

After reading this chapter you'll know what errors to keep an eye out for, and how to ensure you're receiving the most accurate diagnosis possible.

Similar and Overlapping Conditions

If you're experiencing hyperthyroidism symptoms, you should get thyroid blood tests. However, that doesn't mean you should skip *other* types of testing. There are conditions that cause many of the same symptoms as hypothyroidism, and it's possible that your problems are stemming from one of them. Further, it's possible that you're suffering from hyperthyroidism and some other condition *simultaneously*. Certain conditions not only resemble but frequently coexist with hyperthyroidism, making normally unpleasant symptoms even worse.

Therefore, the next five sections briefly describe common conditions that produce many of the same symptoms as hyperthyroidism. If you find one or more of these conditions fits closely with the problems you've having, don't hesitate to bring it up when you speak with your doctor. Take care to clearly explain which symptoms make you suspicious—your doctor will be more interested in what you're feeling and experiencing, so he can make his own diagnosis—and then ask if he believes it makes sense to test for some other specific condition *in addition* to your thyroid testing.

Further, once your illness has been diagnosed, don't stop there; discuss with your doctor whether there are any aspects of your diet, environment, and lifestyle that might have contributed to its development. Dealing with not only your symptoms but the underlying causes vastly increases your chances of achieving optimum health.

Anxiety

Clinical anxiety is a disorder stemming from problems with brain chemistry. It typically causes many of the same symptoms as hyperthyroidism, including the feeling of being anxious, a rapidly pounding heart, shakiness and tremors, weight loss, insomnia, heated skin, and numbness or tingling in hands and feet.

To discover whether your anxiety originates from your brain or your thyroid, simply have your doctor run thyroid blood tests. If you turn out to have clinical anxiety, it's very treatable via medication and talk therapy. Conversely, if you're hyperthyroid, treatment will make your anxiety fade away...along with symptoms you may not even realize you had until you suddenly feel healthy again.

Irregular Heartbeat

There's a feedback link between your brain and your heart. For example, if you see something threatening, your brain will make your heart beat faster to prepare you for either running or fighting.

What you might not know is that the link goes both ways. If your heart starts beating in an irregular manner, chemicals in your brain will respond by making you feel anxious. Further, in a vicious cycle, your brain will then respond by making your heart beat even faster, and you'll end up with all the symptoms associated with anxiety.

This condition can occur due to *atrial fibrillation,* in which your heart's two upper chambers fall out of sync with its two lower chambers and beat too quickly and erratically. It can also occur due to *mitral valve prolapse,* in which the valve between your left-upper chamber and lower chamber doesn't close properly, leading to your heart racing.

If you have such a problem, your doctor might be able to identify it by simply listening to your heart or performing an electrocardiogram (ECG) test in his office. However, if the problem comes and goes or is a mild case, monitoring for 24 hours or more by experienced cardiologists might be required to spot it.

Adrenal Overactivity

If you have a condition that causes your adrenal glands to produce too much cortisol, such as *Cushing's syndrome* or *pheochromocytoma,* you can experience many of the symptoms of hyperthyroidism, including a rapidly pounding heart, anxiety, shakiness and tremors, weight loss, and bone loss.

For detailed information about adrenal diseases, see Chapter 14.

Bipolar Disorder

The manic side of bipolar disorder can spawn many hyperthyroid symptoms, including abnormal excess energy, racing mind, poor concentration, irritability, anxiety, insomnia, increased sex drive, and weight loss.

If you're bipolar, you're likely to know it, but that doesn't mean you aren't also hyperthyroid. You could have both conditions, with the hyperthyroidism making your manic episodes even more extreme than they would be on their own. The best way to be sure is to have your doctor run thyroid blood tests.

Stimulants and Medications

You could be consuming a stimulant or medicine without realizing it's causing hyperthyroidism symptoms. For example, it's common to do more social coffee drinking as you get older. However, your body's ability to break down caffeine *decreases* with age. Therefore, you might be taking in more caffeine precisely at a time in life when you're least able to tolerate it. The side effects of caffeine overdosing mimic hyperthyroidism: anxiety, panic attacks, irritability, shakiness, racing thoughts, a rapid heartbeat, and insomnia.

Making matters worse, the insomnia can lead you to drink even more coffee the next day to stay awake—leading to increasingly severe hyperthyroidism-like symptoms.

A similar situation exists for other stimulants, including nicotine, weight loss pills, and—on a more extreme scale—illegal drugs such as cocaine and ecstasy.

Some medications also have side effects resembling hyperthyroidism. These include prescription amphetamines, certain allergy pills and decongestants, certain antidepressants, and attention deficit disorder with hyperactivity (ADHD) suppressors such as Adderall and Ritalin. The side effects can include anxiety, panic attacks, tremors, rapid heartbeat, numbness or tingling in the hands and feet, insomnia, diarrhea, increased sex drive, and weight loss.

If you suspect an optional stimulant might be causing your problems, simply stop consuming it for a month or two and see if the symptoms disappear.

Alternatively, if you suspect a necessary medication might be the culprit, discuss with your doctor whether you can either use a substitute with less severe side effects or add in other medications that mitigate the side effects.

Key Blood Tests for Hyperthyroidism

The perfect way to detect thyroid disease would be to measure how T3 is affecting the energy levels of your cells' mitochondria (see Chapter 1). If your mitochondria turned out to be supercharged beyond healthy limits, that would be definitive proof you're hyperthyroid.

Unfortunately, medical science currently can't check your energy at the cellular level. So instead of one straightforward test, a doctor who's a thyroid expert will order four types of indirect tests: *TSH, free T4, free T3*, and *antibodies.*

No single test tells the whole story. But if a doctor is experienced at analyzing the results from all of these tests combined and pays attention to your symptoms at the same time, the chances are great that she'll be able to determine whether you're hyperthyroid and what sort of treatment you need.

If you're already on thyroid medication, and/or if you're taking other prescription medications or over-the-counter supplements, schedule your doctor's appointment for the morning and delay taking your pills until after your blood's been extracted. This will decrease the chances of anything skewing your test results.

TSH

As explained in Chapter 1, your thyroid increases and decreases its hormone production based on the orders it receives from a small organ just above your sinuses called the pituitary gland. When your body is low on energy, your pituitary gland responds by making thyroid stimulating hormone, or TSH. This stimulates your thyroid to produce its hormones.

Labs can detect the level of TSH in your bloodstream. When your TSH is below normal, it means your body has too much T4 and T3, and in response, your pituitary gland is holding back its TSH to tell your thyroid to slow down or stop production.

Conversely, when your TSH is above normal, it means you don't have enough T4 and T3, and in response, your pituitary gland is releasing a large amount of TSH to tell your thyroid to step up production.

In other words, there's an inverse relationship between your TSH and thyroid hormone levels because your pituitary gland is continually trying to address any imbalance.

At first blush, it might seem that the TSH test will tell you everything you need to know. In fact, many doctors mistakenly order this test exclusively to check on your thyroid. But relying on TSH alone is a serious mistake for several reasons.

First, the TSH level in your bloodstream isn't a snapshot of your current condition. Instead, it represents a 2–3-month average of your pituitary gland's activities. That's good in that it provides a long-term look at your body. However, it means you can experience hyperthyroid symptoms for some time before your condition is fully reflected by the TSH test. This can lead to a doctor pronouncing you normal when you're really in the early stages of hyperthyroidism.

Further, if you have a back-and-forth condition such as Hashitoxicosis (see Chapter 10), you might swing between hyperthyroidism and hypothyroidism. Because the TSH is a long-term average, the two extremes can cancel each other out, resulting in a TSH level that's normal...and that's masking the war occurring between your immune system and your thyroid.

In addition, the TSH level doesn't reflect whether your thyroid hormones are successfully energizing your cells. For example, if you have an excessive amount of T4 that's not being converted to T3 (see Chapter 1), or if the T3 can't penetrate your cells (see Chapter 14), your TSH level will indicate you're hyperthyroid when you're actually hypothyroid.

Then again, you could have a healthy thyroid but an ailing pituitary gland. For example, if your pituitary has grown a TSH-secreting adenoma (see Chapter 10), it'll cause your thyroid to overproduce hormones, but the high TSH level will make your doctor think that you have the opposite problem and are hypothyroid.

So while the TSH test is a very useful tool, it's not enough by itself to evaluate your status.

Free T4 and Free T3

As explained in Chapter 1, roughly 85–90 percent of the hormones made by your thyroid are T4. T4 is a "storage" hormone designed to circulate in your bloodstream, and be stored in your tissues until thyroid hormone is needed by an area of your body. When energy is called for, your body converts T4 to T3. And it's T3 that does the work of powering up the mitochondria in your cells.

Labs can easily measure the amount of T4 in your bloodstream that's available for conversion, called *free T4* and the amount of circulating T3 that's available for immediate use, called *free T3*.

And unlike the TSH test, which reflects a 2–3-month average, the free T4 and free T3 tests reflect the activities of those hormones within the past week or so. Therefore, these tests offer a more immediate picture of what's happening in your body.

Evaluating your TSH level in conjunction with free T4 and free T3 levels provides a much clearer view than can be gotten from considering TSH alone.

For example, if your thyroid hormone levels changed significantly within the past week, that probably won't turn up in the 2–3 month average represented by your TSH, but it will in your free T4/T3 numbers.

As another example, if your pituitary gland is overactive, your TSH level will be high, making you appear hypothyroid. However, if your free T4/T3 is *also* high, an experienced thyroid doctor will know to suspect a pituitary problem and prescribe an MRI to take a close look at that gland.

If your doctor tests your blood for TSH, free T4, and free T3, the results will provide a pretty good view of your thyroid's status. However, there's one other test category needed to complete the picture.

Antibodies

As explained in Chapters 5 and 10, over 80 percent of all thyroid problems are caused by the autoimmune diseases Hashimoto's (for hypothyroidism) and Graves' (for hyperthyroidism).

Hashimoto's occurs when your immune system attacks your thyroid with thyroid peroxidase (TPO) antibodies and/or thyroglobulin (Tg) antibodies. Initially, these antibodies can swing you back and forth between hyperthyroidism and hypothyroidism, but ultimately, they'll make you hypothyroid.

Graves' occurs when your thyroid is attacked with thyroid stimulating immunoglobulin, or TSI. The antibodies TPO and Tg may also be involved, but what really matters is the TSI. That's because TPO and Tg attack proteins in your thyroid, and their only effect is to destroy the cells. However, TSI binds with the portion of the cells called *receptors* that receive your pituitary glands' TSH. Very much like TSH, the TSI stimulates the cells to produce more hormones, and this overproduction is what makes you hyperthyroid.

If your doctor runs tests only for TSH, T4, and T3, she won't have enough information to determine whether you have Graves' disease, Hashimoto's during a hyperthyroid cycle, or some form of hyperthyroidism that isn't autoimmune at all. Such information is vital in choosing the best method for treating you.

Alternatively, if you're in the preliminary stages of Graves', your TSH, T4, and T3 might all be normal; but TSI testing is likely to turn up the presence of the antibodies, providing you and your doctor with an early warning and the opportunity for preemptive treatment. So when you're being evaluated for the first time for possible hyperthyroidism, your doctor should include antibody tests for TPO, Tg, and (especially) TSI.

If the lab results show high levels of TPO and/or Tg antibodies alone, you probably have Hashimoto's and require treatment for hypothyroidism. But if they show high levels of TSI, you have Graves' and require treatment for that particular form of hyperthyroidism.

Other Testing

As the first section of this chapter indicated, even if your symptoms point strongly to hyperthyroidism, you shouldn't hesitate to allow your doctor to test for other causes. It's possible some other disease is responsible. And it's just as possible that you're hyperthyroid and have another condition occurring at the same time, making your life doubly difficult.

In addition, you might require examination that goes beyond blood tests. For example, if your doctor wants to confirm that you have Graves' disease, he might request an ultrasound to see whether your thyroid shows signs of enlarging as a result of TSI overstimulation.

Another common diagnostic tool is an *iodine uptake and thyroid scan.* For this procedure, your doctor injects you with or has you swallow a tiny amount of radioactive iodine, waits 6–24 hours, and then scans your neck to get a clear picture of what's going on inside it. If the resulting images show even, diffuse enlargement of your thyroid, you probably have Graves' disease. If the iodine concentrates in a few areas of your thyroid, that indicates the toxic nodules of Plummer's disease. Then again, if there are areas of your thyroid that don't absorb the iodine at all, that's reason to suspect thyroid cancer, in which case, the next step should be a biopsy (see Chapter 13).

No matter what the results from the lab are, always pay attention to your symptoms. If your body is sending you messages and your test results don't reflect them, then the problem is usually with the testing, not with what you're feeling.

Analyzing Your Test Results

A few days after your doctor sends your blood to a lab, the test results—which are typically a small collection of numbers fitting onto a single sheet of paper—will be transmitted to her office. As explained in Chapter 4, you can request that her office email or fax that same one-page report to you. You can then study the results at your leisure before the next visit to your doctor. This will allow you to know what to expect, and to prepare any pertinent questions.

Alternatively, you can request a photocopy of the results be mailed to you, or you can pick it up at your doctor's office. Being able to see the precise numbers will empower you to know exactly where you're at, help you more clearly understand how your doctor arrived at her diagnosis, and allow you to double-check your doctor's conclusions.

Whenever you receive test results, first check to make sure they include your correct name and birthdate. Both labs and doctors' offices handle thousands of patients, and mistakes happen.

Each of your tests will result in a single number that's judged by where it falls within the range considered normal for that test. The key thyroid tests and their ranges are as follows:

Key Tests and Ranges for Hyperthyroidism

Test name	Typical lab range	Optimal range
TSH	0.4–4.5 mIU/L	0.3–2.0 mIU/L
Free T4	0.8–1.8 ng/dL	1.1–1.8 ng/dL
Free T3	230–420 pg/dL	same as lab
Thyroid Peroxidase (TPO) Antibodies	<35 IU/mL	same as lab
Thyroglobulin (Tg) Antibodies	<20 IU/mL	same as lab
TSI (TSI) Antibodies	<125% activity	same as lab

Interpreting results using these ranges is mostly straightforward. For example, if your free T3 level is 300 pg/dL (picograms per deciliter of blood), then it's normal because it falls within the range of 230–420 pg/dL. Alternatively, if your T3 level is 700 pg/dL, then it's much too high and you're probably hyperthyroid.

Similarly, if your TPO antibody count is 900 IU/mL (international unit for antibodies per milliliter of blood), that's way over the normal limit of 35 IU/mL and indicates your thyroid is under attack.

A bit more complicated is the range for TSI antibodies. TSI measures how effectively antibodies in your blood bind to cell receptors in the organ of a lab rodent.

This is calculated as a percentage, with anything below 125 percent considered as being within normal range.

"Normal" is misleading in this case, though. If you're at no risk for hyperthyroidism, your TSI score should be below 2 percent—that is, at or close to zero. If your level is between 2 percent and 125 percent, it means you might be on the path to Graves' disease. In this case, it's wise to start taking preventive measures to keep your TSI low, such as reducing your iodine consumption to the safe range of 50–199 mcg per day (see Chapter 18) and avoiding toxins (see Chapter 20). If your TSI level remains below 125 percent, you're unlikely to develop hyperthyroidism symptoms.

When the TSI test reports you have antibodies, it's almost always accurate. When it doesn't, however, there's a 10–20 percent chance your thyroid is being attacked by a form of stimulating antibody that this test just doesn't happen to detect. If your TSI results are under 125 percent but you still suspect you have Graves', you can ask your doctor to focus on other evidence, including low TSH, high T4 and T3, eye problems, and ultrasound and/or thyroid scan tests that show diffuse enlargement of the thyroid.

One other complication with thyroid lab tests is interpreting TSH and free T4 results, because there's a discrepancy between the lab's recommended ranges and what thyroid experts believe is the actual range for good health. If your tests show you're hyperthyroid, you don't have to worry about this. Otherwise, see the "Why 'Normal' Results Might Be Wrong" section in Chapter 7.

Analyzing Patient Test Results

Understanding how to analyze your own test results can be easier after examining real-life examples. The following are true stories of people who were tested for hyperthyroidism and, thanks to their being given the right combination of tests and the right interpretation of the results, were successfully diagnosed and treated.

For each patient, you'll see the test results first. Try to analyze the numbers, and then read the patient's tale to find out if you've interpreted them correctly.

Anxiety

Test name	In range	Out of range	Lab range	Optimal range
TSH	0.8 mIU/L		0.4–4.5 mIU/L	0.3–2.0 mIU/L
Free T4		2.9 ng/dL	0.8–1.8 ng/dL	1.1–1.8 ng/dL
Free T3	290 pg/dL		230–420 pg/dL	same as lab
TPO Antibodies	6 IU/mL		<35 IU/mL	same as lab
Tg Antibodies		>1,000 IU/mL	<20 IU/mL	same as lab
TSI Antibodies	0%		<125%	same as lab

Debbie came to see me in a state of frustration. When she turned 40 a year earlier, she was struck out of the blue with severe anxiety. She'd been to four doctors, and none of them offered a satisfying explanation or successful treatment. Each of them simply indicated she must be "wired" for clinical anxiety. "It's ridiculous," Debbie told me. "I'm the most mellow, low-stress person you could imagine."

As we talked, I learned Debbie's older sister also developed anxiety after turning 40. Her sister was diagnosed with Graves' disease, and after it was treated the problem went away.

Each of the previous doctors has tested Debbie's TSH, found it within the normal range, and dismissed thyroid disease as a possible cause. However, none of them had looked beyond TSH.

I ordered a full range of thyroid blood tests for Debbie. As you can see, her TSH was indeed in the normal range. However, her free T4 was elevated and her Tg antibody count was so high that it was off the charts. That meant Debbie's thyroid was under attack.

Debbie tested negative for TSI, which indicated she didn't have Graves' disease. The TSI test can miss antibodies 10–20 percent of the time, but in this case, the negative result made sense.

Considering the normal TSH level, I was pretty sure Debbie was suffering from Hashitoxicosis, an early stage of Hashimoto's disease that swings a patient between hyperthyroid and hypothyroid states. Because the TSH level is a three-month average, the extreme highs and lows tend to cancel each other out, resulting in a TSH that appears normal.

I ordered an ultrasound test to confirm my diagnosis. The images of Debbie's thyroid showed precisely the damage I expected from Hashitoxicosis.

I treated Debbie for both the hyperthyroid and hypothyroid aspects of her disease, which eased her anxiety. Eventually, Debbie's condition settled into classic hypothyroidism on its own, which was easily treated with thyroid medication.

Lump in the Neck

Test name	In range	Out of range	Lab range	Optimal range
TSH		<0.01 mIU/L	0.4–4.5 mIU/L	0.3–2.0 mIU/L
Free T4		2.4 ng/dL	0.8–1.8 ng/dL	1.1–1.8 ng/dL
Free T3		540 pg/dL	230–420 pg/dL	same as lab
TPO Antibodies	7 IU/mL		<35 IU/mL	same as lab
Tg Antibodies	3 IU/mL		<20 IU/mL	same as lab
TSI Antibodies		158%	<125%	same as lab

Angie had a clearly visible growth in her neck. "It's been there a while," she said. "I didn't come in sooner because I was terrified it's cancer. And I still am, but ignoring it hasn't kept it from growing bigger." I assured her that a lot of people react the same way, and that I'd do my best for her no matter what it was.

I gave Angie a brief physical exam, and found the lump was on her thyroid. I asked Angie if she'd noticed anything else unusual. "I'm embarrassed to say this," she replied, "but over the last six months I've been sweating like a geyser from my hands, feet, underarms, and the back of my head." I ran through a symptoms checklist with her, and discovered that she had a strong appetite but was continually losing weight: "My friends say it looks like I'm wasting away. It's another reason I fear it's cancer."

"Angie, does the lump hurt?" I asked. "Sometimes," she said. "And I'm finding it harder to swallow."

"That's good news," I said, "because cancer usually doesn't hurt. And your collection of symptoms makes me suspect another cause. Let's run some tests."

As you can see, Angie's TSH level was an off-the-charts at <0.01. This meant her pituitary gland had essentially shut down its TSH production. She also had high levels of T4 and T3, and TSI antibodies. It was a classic case of Graves' disease, complete with goiter.

I prescribed 10 mg daily of Tapazole (see Chapter 12) to manage Angie's hyperthyroidism. That was just enough to make her symptoms tolerable but not enough to raise her TSH level. Keeping Angie's TSH low discouraged her thyroid from creating new cells for her goiter. Because the current cells died out without being replaced, the goiter shrank naturally over the next year until its size was insignificant.

Angie and I had to continue keeping her TSH low so the goiter wouldn't grow back, but after another year on the Tapazole, her Graves' disease petered out, allowing Angie to enjoy normal thyroid function again.

Keeping Her Baby Healthy

Test name	In range	Out of range	Lab range	Optimal range
TSH		<0.01 mIU/L	0.4–4.5 mIU/L	0.3–2.0 mIU/L
Free T4		2.9 ng/dL	0.8–1.8 ng/dL	1.1–1.8 ng/dL
Free T3		500 pg/dL	230–420 pg/dL	same as lab
TPO Antibodies	11 IU/mL		<35 IU/mL	same as lab
Tg Antibodies	2 IU/mL		<20 IU/mL	same as lab
TSI Antibodies		180%	<125%	same as lab

Because of its hormonal upheavals, pregnancy is sometimes the trigger for thyroid disease. That's why good obstetricians periodically run blood tests to check for such occurrences. And that's how Sally discovered, near the end of her first trimester, that her TSH level was an off-the-charts at <0.01, indicating thyroid hormone levels so high that the pituitary gland had stopped producing TSH.

Sally's obstetrician referred her to me. While I examined Sally, we chatted. "I've been feeling anxious," she said, "and my heart has been beating super-fast, but this is my first baby. I just assumed it was all part of being pregnant."

After hearing this, I took Sally's blood and ordered a full range of thyroid tests. As you can see, Sally turned out to have high levels of T4, T3, and TSI antibodies, which meant she had Graves' disease. I followed up with an ultrasound, which confirmed the diagnosis via images of an enlarged thyroid.

I explained to Sally that treatment was especially important in her case because Graves' posed a risk for a miscarriage, birth defects, and heart damage. There was also a risk of the disease spreading to her baby unless we got it under control.

I put Sally on a 2-month starting dose of PTU (see Chapter 12). This lowered Sally's T4 and T3 into the normal range, but her TSI remained at 180 percent. I countered with a gentle increase in the PTU dosage. I was relieved six weeks later when Sally's TSI came down to 75 percent. I kept Sally at the same dosage for the remainder of her pregnancy. She had a beautiful baby boy, with no complications.

Over the Counter

Test name	In range	Out of range	Lab range	Optimal range
TSH		0.04 mIU/L	0.4–4.5 mIU/L	0.3–2.0 mIU/L
Free T4		4.2 ng/dL	0.8–1.8 ng/dL	1.1–1.8 ng/dL
Free T3		670 pg/dL	230–420 pg/dL	same as lab
TPO Antibodies	0 IU/mL		<35 IU/mL	same as lab
Tg Antibodies	3 IU/mL		<20 IU/mL	same as lab
TSI Antibodies	1%		<125%	same as lab

Leonard was a charming gentleman in his 60s who loved to talk about diet and supplements and took dozens of over-the-counter medications.

Leonard came to me because both of his hands had developed tremors over the past year, and the condition was growing worse. While we talked, I learned that Leonard was also experiencing a rapid heartbeat and trouble sleeping.

I ran a battery of tests. The most significant results were his thyroid blood test numbers: a low TSH, and very high T4 and T3.

I remembered Leonard's over-the-counter pills, and asked him to bring them all in for me to examine. One of the bottles was for weight loss, and it listed "lyophilized bovine thyroid extract" as an ingredient. The active hormones of non-prescription supplements are supposed to be removed before they're sold. However, these drugs aren't carefully monitored, and accidents happen. Leonard took four of these pills three times daily. Considering he had no anti-body activity, I was pretty sure Leonard's over-the-counter meds were behind his hyperthyroidism.

I advised Leonard to stop taking his weight-loss pills (which weren't good for him anyway). After four months, Leonard's TSH, T4, and T3 returned to normal, his tremors went away, his heart rate quieted down, and he once again slept soundly.

If you've been diagnosed as having hyperthyroidism, you're ready to be treated. The steps for getting you well again are covered next.

CHAPTER 12

Treating Hyperthyroidism

For those who are hypothyroid, treatment is relatively easy; all that's required are pills supplying the hormones they're missing. Because these are the same hormones normally made by the thyroid, their bodies simply welcome the boost the medication provides.

But if you've been diagnosed as hyperthyroid, you effectively need to combat your body's natural ability to produce thyroid hormones, which is a trickier process. It can be successfully achieved via low-impact remedies, antithyroid medication, radioactive iodine, and/or surgery—and the help of an experienced doctor who carefully monitors your progress.

This chapter will guide you through the options, so you can make the best choices for your long-term health.

Low-Impact Remedies

If you get tested as soon as you notice hyperthyroidism symptoms, the disease might be detected at a sufficiently early stage for your excess T4 and T3 levels to be relatively mild. This doesn't occur often with Graves' disease, but it does with other forms of hyperthyroidism such as Plummer's. If you're being treated by a doctor familiar with natural medicine, identifying your condition early on provides an opportunity to try gentle remedies to keep the hyperthyroidism from becoming worse.

The advantages to this approach are that the risks of side effects are near zero, and it'll cost much less than prescription medication. If your condition can be stabilized, you might be able to stay on the nonintrusive treatment until it either ends the disease and restores you to full health, or maintains you at relatively safe hormone levels until the disease burns itself out over 2–3 years. At the end of this process, your thyroid might return to normal, or you might become hypothyroid, in which case, you'd start taking thyroid medication (see Chapters 8 and 9).

Dietary Changes

Many patients have found that switching to a vegan or vegan-like diet for about 3–6 months either mitigates or ends their thyroid disease. Studies have confirmed this for hypothyroidism. Research results have been more mixed for hyperthyroidism, but in my experience, dietary changes tend to be effective for both conditions.

Changing lifelong eating habits isn't easy. But if you can manage to spend 3–6 months on a diet of fruits, vegetables, nuts, seeds, beans, legumes, and gluten-free grains, it might have a huge positive impact on your hyperthyroidism. For much more about this, see Chapter 18.

Anti-Infection Supplements

Just in case your thyroid issue is at least partially being caused by an infection, consider trying over-the-counter antiviral/antibacterial supplements to see if they make you feel better. Popular supplements include vitamin C (1,000–2,000 mg, taken with food to avoid upsetting your stomach), cat's claw, L-lysine, lemon balm, and goldenseal (taken at the dosages recommended on their respective labels).

Fluoride

Fluoride is famous for fighting tooth decay. However, it can also combat hyperthyroidism. That's because your thyroid's hormone production is dependent on iodine, and fluoride's chemical composition is so similar to iodine that your thyroid can't tell the difference between the two. Your thyroid will therefore absorb any fluoride in your bloodstream. The more fluoride your thyroid takes in, the less room there is for iodine, and the more likely it is that the fluoride will block iodine from your thyroid's hormone construction sites. The result is a substantial reduction in thyroid hormones.

The level of fluoride in toothpaste, or that's added to the water supply of many communities, is too low to affect your thyroid. But in a more concentrated form, fluoride is an effective suppressor of T4 and T3 overproduction.

Fluoride was frequently used to treat hyperthyroidism in the past. It isn't anymore, possibly because there's no financial incentive for drug companies to champion its use when there are much more expensive alternatives. But if you can find a doctor who'll agree to monitor its use, you'll discover fluoride can be purchased cheaply from virtually any drugstore and is available in numerous forms (chewable tablets, gels, lozenges, etc.).

If your hyperthyroidism is mild, you might first opt for the dietary changes in Chapter 18 and see if they end your hyperthyroidism symptoms on their own.

If you and your doctor decide you need more help, though, fluoride typically causes no complications in moderate dosages.

While You're Waiting...

Low-impact remedies can be very effective, but you must be patient to experience their effects. That's because your thyroid has already made and stored a large amount of its hormones, and it'll take 4–6 weeks for those existing supplies to be used up. All the remedies can do is reduce the subsequent number of hormones your thyroid produces. You should therefore allow for 4–6 weeks before noticing a difference in how you feel.

That doesn't mean you need to suffer while you wait, though. You can, and should, take steps to manage your symptoms. You can use prescription medication to do this, and options are described later in this chapter. But natural remedies are available for this purpose as well.

For example, you can typically slow down your heart rate by consuming more magnesium. You can do this, in part, by eating magnesium-rich foods, such as legumes (adzuki beans, black beans), dark green vegetables (broccoli, organic kale and spinach), and nuts and seeds (almonds, cashews, pumpkin seeds).

It also helps to cut out caffeinated beverages, such as coffee and soda, as they both reduce magnesium and raise your heart rate.

And if you're experiencing anxiety, you might be able to calm it with theanine, an amino acid commonly present in tea (and one of the reasons people find tea soothing). You might also benefit from kava-kava, a beverage made from the plant of the same name, which relaxes without affecting mental clarity.

Prescription Medications

The primary medication for treating hyperthyroidism is *Tapazole*. There's also a generic version called *methimazole*.

A secondary option is *propylthiouracil (PTU)*, or *PTU*. PTU is an older drug, and it's available as a generic exclusively (there's no branded version).

Tapazole and PTU are called antithyroid medications because they work by fighting against your thyroid's natural functions. Specifically, they disrupt the process your thyroid uses to turn iodine into hormones. They're very effective at reducing T4 and T3 production, regardless of the form and severity of your hyperthyroidism.

Therefore, if your condition has gotten beyond the early, mild stage described in the previous section, these medications are typically your best choice for managing your hyperthyroidism (along with the dietary changes recommended in Chapter 18, which are worth trying at any stage of the disease).

Once your condition is stabilized, you can usually stay on the medication until the disease runs its course over 2–3 years. At that point your thyroid might return to normal; or you might become hypothyroid and simply go on thyroid medication.

Tapazole vs. PTU

Tapazole has several highly significant advantages over PTU:

O It produces results faster, typically returning your hormone levels to normal in 4–6 weeks. PTU can take 3–4 months to do the same thing.

O It needs to be taken only once a day. PTU must be taken two or three times a day.

O It will have virtually no effect on any subsequent attempt for treatment using radioactive iodine. PTU reduces the odds of subsequent radiation being effective.

O It has fewer serious side effects.

You'd typically turn to PTU if you were allergic to Tapazole or found Tapazole to be ineffective for you. PTU is also preferable for treating Graves' disease during the first trimester of pregnancy, because Tapazole has a greater chance of causing birth defects during the first three months of fetal development. Otherwise, Tapazole is the best treatment choice for most people.

Tapazole and PTU Side Effects

Both Tapazole and PTU share some side effects. When taking either of them, there's up to a 13 percent chance you'll experience itching, rash, hives, joint pain, arthritis, fever, abnormal taste sensations, nausea, or vomiting.

There's also a tiny (0.2–0.5 percent) chance of developing *agranulocytosis,* which causes a reduction in the white blood cells that fight infection—and a very serious chink in the armor of your immune system. Your doctor should periodically test for this. Further, if you get a sore throat or other infection while on either medication, see your doctor right away so she can run a white cell count on your blood, and don't take the medication again until the lab results arrive and show that you're okay.

In addition, PTU has one major side effect that resulted in a 2009 FDA warning: the potential to cause severe liver damage. While this rarely occurs, when it happens it can completely shut down the liver, and it's led to 13 deaths and 11 liver transplants to date. That means if you're on PTU, both you and your doctor need to pay special attention for telltale signs of liver problems, such as a yellowish tinge to the skin or eyes.

Doctors who favor radioactive iodine as a first-line treatment for hyperthyroidism point to PTU's drawbacks, arguing radiation is a more convenient and safer approach. And in this case, a reasonable argument can be made.

When it comes to Tapazole, however, it's been my experience that if you have a knowledgeable doctor to monitor you, using this medication creates few complications, and its benefits far outweigh the risks.

Natural versus prescription medication doesn't have to be an either/or choice. Most of my patients do extremely well starting off on low to moderate doses of Tapazole (prescription medication) in combination with fluoride (a low-impact remedy). After a few months, I'm able to wean most of them off the Tapazole, at which point they do fine on the fluoride alone—which is inexpensive and has almost no side effects in moderate doses.

Other Medications

While both Tapazole and PTU are very effective, they take a while to kick in. As mentioned previously, you must wait 4–6 weeks to improve on Tapazole and 3–4 months on PTU.

Further, your doctor might decide to put you on a dosage of medication that keeps you marginally hyperthyroid. This is often a good strategy if you have one or more goiters, because your TSH must remain low for the goiters to shrink. But it means you'll still have some remaining symptoms.

Then again, you might be allergic to both Tapazole and PTU. In this case, you'll want some help getting through each day until you're ready for either radioactive iodine treatment or surgery.

In all such situations, you'll require medications to suppress key hyperthyroid problems. Most commonly, you'll need to lower your heart rate. This can be accomplished by a *beta blocker*, which is a drug that blocks the effects of adrenaline, making your heart beat more slowly and with less force. It also helps reduce your blood pressure and improve your blood's circulation. The best beta blockers for hyperthyroidism include *atenolol* and *propranolol*.

Block-and-Replace Therapy

If you're on antithyroid medication such as Tapazole, your doctor will monitor you via periodic checkups for 2–3 years until your hyperthyroidism starts petering out on its own. Your doctor will then gradually withdraw your treatment as your thyroid hormone levels lower.

At that point either your thyroid will return to normal, in which case you're home free; or your levels will continue falling, making you hypothyroid.

If it becomes clear you're heading in the latter direction, an experienced doctor won't just withdraw treatment and let you plummet into hypothyroidism. Instead, she'll start putting you on low doses of thyroid hormones while you're still being treated for hyperthyroidism.

I call this "driving with the parking brake on," because it allows your doctor to control how quickly you're moving in both directions. It ensures your T4 and T3 levels don't jump up again, while at the same time gently eases you into your new hypothyroid state. It's officially called *block-and-replace therapy* because your doctor is blocking the disease while she's replacing any lack of hormones.

After several months or so, your doctor can stop the antithyroid medication entirely and simply treat you for being hypothyroid. The latter is a cause for celebration because it essentially means you're out of danger. Once you're hypo-thyroid, all you must do is take thyroid medication every morning to maintain healthy hormone levels.

Some doctors are so enthusiastic about block-and-replace therapy that they advocate using it for the entire medication process. Studies don't support this view, though; while it does no harm, this approach doesn't shorten the duration of treatment or improve the outcome. That said, if your T4/T3 levels are continually fluctuating between being too high and too low, block-and-replace therapy is typically the perfect solution.

Radiation and Surgery

Most doctors in Europe greatly prefer using medication to treat hyperthyroidism. In America, however, the first choice of most doctors is *radioiodine ablation*. This uses radioactive iodine to destroy a substantial percentage of the thyroid's cells, making it too small to overproduce hormones.

This works because the thyroid is the only gland in your body that absorbs iodine. When you're given iodine that's radioactive (via pill or injection), the iodine will be ignored by the rest of your body and travel straight to your throat, where it'll be eagerly absorbed by your thyroid cells. The radiation will then kill off the cells.

If your doctor recommends this strategy, he'll probably tell you that there's no risk of developing cancer from it. However, a major study of 2,500 patients followed over 10 years (through 2002) concluded that those who underwent this procedure were later struck by cancer at a 20 percent higher rate than those who didn't. That's a highly significant difference.

Another disadvantage is that your doctor will err on the side of making you hypo-thyroid. While that's a much safer condition than hyperthyroidism, it's not as good as returning to normal thyroid function; and the latter happens as much as 70 percent of the time for those who choose the medication route.

On the positive side, radioiodine ablation takes 6–18 weeks, while it typically takes 2–3 years of medication and skilled monitoring by your doctor to manage your hyperthyroidism until the disease ends itself naturally.

In addition, radioiodine ablation is a tremendously useful option if you're allergic to Tapazole, or if Tapazole simply doesn't happen to work for you.

I've found some patients like the apparent finality of radiation over the gradual monitoring and adjustment process of medication. In practice, however, for roughly 1 out of 5 patients radioiodine ablations won't work the first time, requiring a second dose...and further increasing the risk of cancer down the line.

In most cases, I prefer the medication route for my patients. I find it works with few complications, and it creates no further risk of cancer. But both approaches have positives and negatives.

Finally, you have the option of getting half or all of your thyroid surgically removed. This is considered a last resort, however. While an operation will end your hyperthyroidism, it risks doing damage to your parathyroid glands and vocal cord nerves (see Chapter 13).

Hyperthyroid Patient Stories

It can be easier to understand treatment options when they're viewed within the context of people's lives. The following are true stories of patients who were struggling with hyperthyroidism. They were all restored to full health via medication.

Weary of Radiation

Martha had undergone radioiodine ablation treatment for her Graves' disease...twice. She was still hyperthyroid.

About 20 percent of patients must return for a second dose of radiation before their T4 and T3 levels fall to normal or hypothyroid levels. A second treatment not being enough either was unusual, though. I didn't blame Martha for being frustrated. Further, her doctor was now recommending surgery. Concerned about the risk of complications, she sought me out for a fresh perspective.

Martha was stable on high doses of both Tapazole and the beta blocker atenolol. I told her I'd like to try a slightly different approach for a month and see what happened. After she agreed, I kept Martha on her current medications but added low doses of fluoride (to block iodine) and lithium (to ease her anxiety). On her first retest, Martha's T4 and T3 levels were in the normal range for the first time in years. She also felt much less anxious.

We moved forward with a medicine-based treatment. Martha continued to improve, and we were able to lower her dosages over the next several months while keeping her T4/T3 levels steady.

Thyroid-Blocking Medication

Rebecca had a severe case of Graves' disease. Her TSH was an off-the-charts <0.01 mIU/L, and her free T4 was a sky-high 5.9 ng/dL. I explained that managing her hyperthyroidism would be like stopping a train. It would take the strength of Superman to abruptly bring it to a halt, but after that a simple wheel chock could hold it in place.

I prescribed a high daily dose of 60 mg of Tapazole over the first six weeks to slow down the disease. After that, I was able to bring the daily dosage down to 10 mg for maintenance. Soon she was managed on desiccated thyroid medication.

Block and Replace

Peter came to see me for management of his Plummer's disease after unceasing anxiety and panic attacks. His previous doctor had prescribed 20 mg of Tapazole daily, which ended up making Peter hypothyroid. His doctor then prescribed a low dose of Synthroid, which made the hyperthyroidism come back worse than ever.

Afraid of getting even worse, Peter did nothing for six months. Then the misery of his symptoms led him to seek me out for a second opinion. Considering his experiences, I told Peter he'd probably do well on block-and-replace therapy. I prescribed 5 mg of Tapazole and 75 mcg of Synthroid. Within a month, Peter told me he felt like himself again.

Over the following months, we made minor adjustments. After Peter had been stable for a full year, I very gradually tapered him off both the Tapazole and Synthroid. He remained healthy. I have Peter keeping a sharp eye out for symptoms, though, and schedule him to see me every six months, just in case there's a recurrence.

Hyperthyroidism is a serious disease, and can be scary. But if you take the right steps, it's highly treatable.

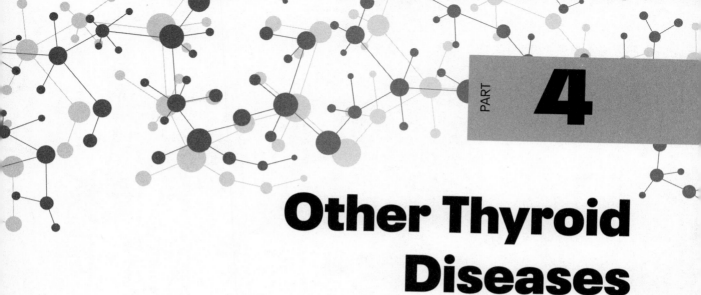

PART 4

Other Thyroid Diseases

In this part, Chapter 13 provides a step-by-step guide to diagnosing and treating thyroid cancer. The key things to remember are that the most common forms of thyroid cancer have a 97 percent cure rate; and that, as John Diamond wrote, "Cancer is a word, not a sentence."

Chapter 14 covers how to identify and treat problems with your thyroid's partners, the adrenal glands. Chapter 15 tells you about other thyroid-related problems, including parathyroid disease, thyroiditis, and MEN syndrome.

One of the most tragic aspects of thyroid disease is the havoc it can play with minds and emotions. Millions of people are suffering from depression, anxiety, and other mental disorders because they don't realize they have a thyroid problem. Chapter 16 explains how to avoid this trap.

And if you're a woman, read Chapter 17 to ensure that thyroid disease doesn't make a tough time worse when you're experiencing PMS, fertility problems, postpartum issues, perimenopause, or menopause.

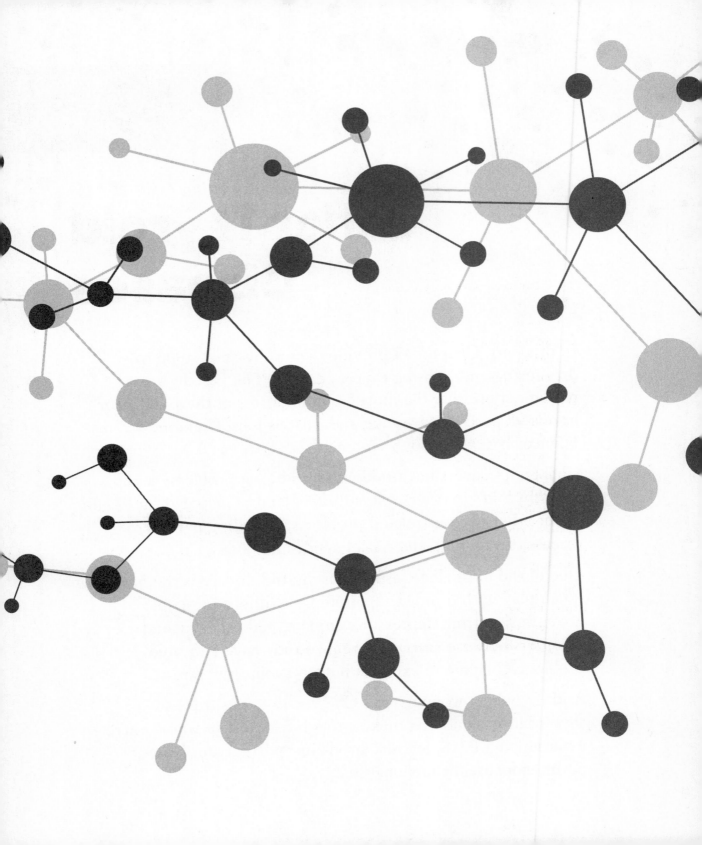

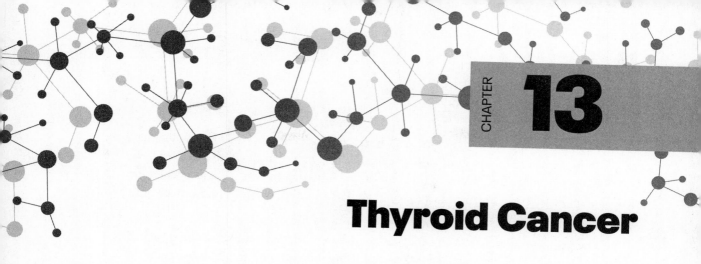

CHAPTER

13

Thyroid Cancer

Cancer is a word, not a sentence.

—John Diamond

One of the scariest words anyone can hear is *cancer*. It's a disease that, like a malicious invader, launches an assault in one area of your body and then keeps expanding its territory, killing everything in its path.

When it comes to thyroid cancer, the good news is that it's rarely fatal. There are around 53,000 cases of thyroid cancer diagnosed in the United States each year, and around 2,200 deaths result from it. The odds for survival are over 95 percent. That's because the most common forms of thyroid cancer grow slowly, and can usually be stopped via surgical removal of one or both of your thyroid's lobes before the cancer spreads to other parts of your body. If only one of your lobes needs to be removed, the other will probably be able to take on the work of producing your thyroid hormones by itself. Alternatively, if the entire thyroid must be removed, your doctors can usually exploit the unique characteristics of thyroid cells to target any remnants of the cancer post-surgery and destroy them.

One of the most challenging aspects of thyroid cancer is dealing with the fear and stress it brings. This chapter will help you understand the process for evaluation and treatment, empowering you to ask the right questions and make the best decisions...and giving you the peace of mind of knowing that the odds are enormously in your favor.

Noticing Nodules

There's a saying among doctors: "If it hurts, it's probably not cancer." You can have thyroid cancer and not know it for years, because you're unlikely to feel it or have it substantially affect your thyroid's ability to function. In fact, it's not unusual for someone to die of unrelated causes and be discovered to have thyroid cancer only upon postmortem examination.

The primary sign of thyroid cancer is one or more masses, called *nodules,* growing on the thyroid. They're typically noticed when one of them grows big enough to be seen or felt through the throat. A nodule might also call attention to itself by growing large enough to give you trouble swallowing, or by pressing on your vocal cord nerves to make your voice hoarse.

By age 50, roughly 50 percent of us have one or more thyroid nodules. More than 95 percent of the time, these nodules are harmless. But when a nodule grows large enough to be noticed, it's important to have a doctor check it out for safety's sake. This is because while thyroid cancer cells typically duplicate themselves slowly, each duplication doubles the size of the mass. It can take decades for a few pioneering cancer cells to duplicate enough times to become a significant nodule; but at that point, even though the rate of duplication remains the same, the doubling effect means the cancer cells have to be dealt with because they might soon spread beyond your thyroid.

So even though the odds are against a nodule being cancerous, the possibility shouldn't be ignored. That's especially the case if you're a woman, as you're three times as likely to develop thyroid cancer as a man; and if you're age 30 or over, as both the risk of having thyroid cancer and its severity increase as you get older.

Taking an Initial Look

There's nothing you can do on your own to evaluate a nodule, so you need to see a doctor. You can start with your general practitioner or go straight to a specialist, which in this case, is an ear, nose, and throat (ENT) surgeon.

Either way, your doctor will typically perform a manual exam, take some blood to send to a lab for thyroid testing, and then prescribe an ultrasound test. You shouldn't hesitate to agree to the latter, as it's relatively quick and inexpensive—and it doesn't involve radiation, so it's entirely safe.

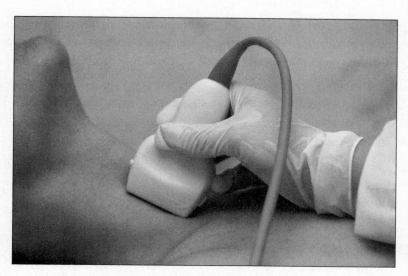

Checking the thyroid via ultrasound
(Licensed from Shutterstock Images)

An ultrasound lets your doctor see what's going on inside your throat by bouncing high-frequency sound waves off your thyroid (like how bats and submarines use sound to navigate). A technician will lubricate your throat with jelly to make the sound waves transmit more effectively, then move a handheld component of the machine over your throat to take pictures of your thyroid, including its nodules.

A specialist will then examine the images, looking for such details as whether a nodule is entirely filled with fluid (in which case, it might be a mere cyst), if it's one of a number of nodules the same size (which could mean you have a benign multi-nodule goiter), or if it's solid and attached to an unusually large number of veins (which is cause for suspicion because cancer is greedy for blood, forming new blood vessels just to feed itself).

Alternatively, if your doctor suspects you're hyperthyroid, he might prescribe an iodine uptake and thyroid scan, which involves your swallowing a tiny amount of radioactive iodine. The radiation will "light up" whatever absorbs it, and the only things in your body that absorb iodine are thyroid cells. If a nodule is causing your hyperthyroidism, it'll show up as "hot," meaning it absorbed the iodine and is probably responsible for your having too many thyroid hormones. If a nodule is "cold," however—meaning it's not absorbing the iodine and is making no hormones—that's cause for suspicion, because some types of cancer cells don't use iodine and produce nothing other than more cancer cells. About 10 percent of "cold" nodules turn out to be cancerous.

If your ultrasound or uptake scan provides enough information to consider your nodule(s) benign, then you can stop exploring the possibility of cancer for now. However, you should see your doctor at least once a year so she can monitor your thyroid and note whether there's any further growth.

On the other hand, if the testing leaves room for suspicion, this is the time to start looking for an ENT surgeon who has long experience and a great reputation for diagnosing and, if necessary, dealing with thyroid cancer.

Getting a Biopsy

The next step in checking your nodule(s) is a *fine needle aspiration biopsy*. This involves your ENT doctor attaching a very thin—and relatively painless—needle to a syringe and sticking it into your throat, aiming for every major nodule on your thyroid (usually based on his feeling its location, or sometimes with the aid of an ultrasound machine).

For each insertion, you'll be asked to hold your breath so your doctor can gently rock the needle back and forth to gather as much tissue as possible. Your doctor will then retract the syringe to capture small bits of tissue from the nodule. He'll repeat this procedure 2–6 times for each large nodule. This is a quick procedure that's usually performed in your doctor's office, and when done properly isn't much more of a bother than getting an injection.

The samples from your biopsy will be sent to a *cytopathologist*, who's an expert at evaluating minute clues about cells. The cytopathologist will carefully examine your samples under a microscope, and will then reach one of four conclusions:

○ You don't have thyroid cancer and your nodule's cells show no signs of cancer. This happens about 70 percent of the time.

○ You do have thyroid cancer and your doctor's needle captured cells that are clearly cancerous. This happens about 5–10 percent of the time.

○ Not enough thyroid tissue was gathered to make an analysis. This happens about 10 percent of the time.

○ No cells were found that are definitively cancerous, but there are cells with suspicious characteristics. This happens about 10–15 percent of the time.

The first three situations are relatively straightforward. If the cytopathologist finds no significant signs of cancer, the chances are over 95 percent that you're fine. Simply be sure to visit your general practitioner every six months to check whether there's been any nodule growth.

Alternatively, if the cytopathologist determines you have cancer, the chances she's right are also more than 95 percent (and if she's highly experienced, closer to 100 percent). This isn't a cause for panic, as most thyroid cancer is as treatable as cancer gets; but it does mean you'll need surgery. (More on this shortly.)

If not enough useable tissue was gathered, then the biopsy must be repeated. This isn't unheard of. However, you might want to have a discussion with your ENT about what went wrong and also casually ask how many thyroid biopsies he's performed. If your doctor hasn't already handled hundreds of thyroid cancer cases, you should seriously consider finding one who has.

The most complicated situation is when the cytopathologist has enough tissue to work with but still can't make a definitive judgment. This can happen for a number of reasons. For example, your doctor might fail to capture cancer cells during any of his needle insertions (a nodule can contain both cancerous and benign cells), but succeed at capturing nearby cells that hint at the presence of cancer. As another example, your doctor might capture only follicular cells. Follicular cancer comprises about 12 percent of all thyroid cancers, but a biopsy is incapable of providing enough information to distinguish between cancerous and non-cancerous follicular cells.

When faced with this kind of gray area, the only way to find out for certain whether a nodule is cancerous is to surgically remove it and place it under a microscope. However, the surgery carries significant risks (described below). And in more than 75 percent of these cases, the nodule turns out to be benign.

At the same time, there's also a risk in letting a nodule that might be cancerous continue to grow...and potentially spread beyond your thyroid. This is a situation in which you want a deeply experienced ENT doctor to advise you. You should ask for a copy of the cytopathologist's report and have your doctor explain the details behind the finding of "indeterminate."

Another pre-surgery test worth asking about is a *coarse needle biopsy*, which allows for the removal of a greater amount of thyroid tissue than fine needle aspiration for nodules three quarters of an inch or larger. Not all doctors are qualified to perform this procedure; but when used as a follow-up for certain types of indeterminate results, coarse needle biopsies have been found to significantly reduce unnecessary thyroid surgeries.

You might also want to get a second opinion. Surgery on your throat isn't something to take lightly, and neither is cancer. Don't hesitate to gather more information before deciding.

Selecting Surgery

If your biopsy showed you have thyroid cancer, or if the results were sufficiently suspicious to justify pursuing a definitive answer, your next step is to have surgery.

If you choose this route, you'll first be placed under anesthesia. Your ENT surgeon will then open your neck and *very* carefully work on your thyroid. This is a delicate procedure because there are some critical body parts nearby. Specifically, nerves involved with your vocal cords and with swallowing are right next to your thyroid. If these nerves are pulled too hard or otherwise injured, it could impair your ability to speak or swallow. The negative results could include a hoarse or whispery voice, with reduced power and/or range. In most cases such issues are temporary, but there are rare instances when the damage is permanent. This is a major reason to choose an ENT who has performed many previous thyroid surgeries.

Also at risk are your *parathyroids*, which are small glands residing behind your thyroid that regulate the amount of calcium in your blood and bones (see Chapter 15). The precise location, number, and size of these glands varies from person to person, increasing the odds of accidentally damaging one or more of them. Thyroid surgeons focus heavily on protecting the parathyroids, so the likelihood of permanent harm is small. But temporary injury is a real possibility, happening to about 8 percent of patients. (A telltale sign is tingling or numbness in your fingers, toes, or lips within the first few days following surgery.) Even if you feel no symptoms, you'll be told to take calcium supplements for a month following the surgery to lighten the strain on your parathyroids in case they need time to recover.

During surgery, your doctor first explores your thyroid to spot all nodules and anything else suspicious. If this inspection makes it apparent that you have cancer on both lobes, then he'll remove the entire thyroid.

Otherwise, the lobe with the largest (or only) nodule is removed first. If you're in a top facility with both a cytopathologist and cytology lab available for the operation—which is ideal—the lobe's cells are examined while you're still under anesthesia. This provides your surgeon with definitive information about whether there's cancer present and, if so, what type of cancer. Your surgeon can then decide whether to remove the rest of your thyroid or to allow the second lobe to remain. In the latter case you'll probably still have a fully functioning thyroid, with the remaining lobe simply doing twice the amount of the work as before.

If your hospital doesn't have the resources to check your thyroid's cells during the operation, though, then your doctor might remove one lobe, end the operation, and wait until a cytopathologist examines the lobe to decide if you need a second operation to take out the rest of your thyroid.

Alternatively, if the results of your biopsy strongly indicate cancer, you and your doctor might decide before the surgery that he'll remove the entire thyroid. This spares you from undergoing a second operation and provides peace of mind that the cancer won't spread—but at the cost of a functioning thyroid that might never become cancerous. The pros and cons of this decision vary depending on such factors as the type of cancer involved (some are more aggressive than others) and your age (thyroid cancer becomes more dangerous as you get older).

Types of Thyroid Cancer

After you've had surgery, sections of your removed nodule(s) will be studied by a cytopathologist to determine precisely what sort of thyroid cancer caused them. This is important information because it'll help determine what additional steps need to be taken.

The primary possibilities are that you don't have cancer, or that you have papillary, follicular, or medullary cancer. (There are other types, but they collectively account for less than 5 percent of thyroid cancer cases.)

No Cancer

After removing half your thyroid, your doctor may find the nodule(s) growing on it to be benign. As mentioned previously, this happens more than 75 percent of the time. You might feel bad about losing a healthy thyroid lobe, as well as risking damage to your parathyroids, and your ability to easily speak and swallow; but you might also feel glad about having the peace of mind of knowing that you're cancer-free.

Either way, you still have half of a functioning thyroid, and there's a good chance it'll make all the thyroid hormones you need. For safety's sake, however, keep a lookout for hypothyroid symptoms (see Chapter 6). Also, take care to get your thyroid hormone levels tested after six months, and then annually, in case you eventually become hypothyroid as a result of your remaining lobe doing twice as much work as it was designed for.

Papillary Cancer

By far the most common form of thyroid cancer is *papillary,* accounting for about 80 percent of cases. Papillary cancer typically stems from exposure to radiation. It's slow growing, taking 10–20 years to develop to the point where it's noticeable.

It's also *well differentiated,* meaning it closely resembles normal thyroid cells. For example, papillary cancer absorbs iodine like a normal thyroid cell—which means it's ideally suited for destruction by radioactive iodine. (See the next section, "Getting Radioactive.")

Papillary cancer tends to stay in the neck—for instance, invading the lymph nodes. However, around 5–10 percent of patients eventually develop papillary cancer in other areas of their bodies, particularly the lungs and bones. So even though it's slow growing, this cancer must be taken seriously and destroyed before it spreads.

Follicular Cancer

Follicular is the second most common form of thyroid cancer, accounting for about 12 percent of cases. Its causes are believed to include radiation, genetics, and low iodine consumption.

Like papillary, follicular cancer is well differentiated, absorbing iodine like normal thyroid cells—which means it's also ideally suited for destruction by radioactive iodine.

Follicular cancer doesn't tend to spread in the neck, but around 20 percent of patients eventually develop it in the lungs and bones.

Medullary Cancer

Medullary is the third most common form of thyroid cancer, accounting for around 5 percent of cases. Its causes are unknown beyond genetics; about 25 percent of people struck by it have a family history of the disease.

Medullary cancer is *not* well differentiated, so it doesn't absorb iodine like a normal thyroid cell and won't be affected by radioactive iodine. It's also not affected by chemotherapy.

Medullary cancer is substantially more aggressive than papillary and follicular, invading lymph nodes over more than 50 percent of the time.

The best method for eliminating medullary cancer is surgery—removing the entire thyroid, possibly the lymph nodes, and anything else it appears to have invaded.

Follow-up visits to check for any recurrence are mandatory. If the cancer comes back, the best option is usually more surgery. However, sometimes radiation can also be effective.

Getting Radioactive

One of the advantages of getting your entire thyroid removed is it makes you a candidate for *radioactive iodine treatment*. This is a clever way to destroy papillary and follicular cancer (making up about 92 percent of thyroid cancer cases) by taking advantage of one of the unique properties of the thyroid.

Specifically, the thyroid is the only gland in your body that absorbs iodine. And although your thyroid was removed, many of its cells are still in your throat... including cancerous ones. To deal with this, you won't be allowed thyroid medication for 4–6 weeks after your surgery. This will put you into a severe hypothyroid state—and starve your thyroid cells of iodine.

You'll then be given a single dose of radioactive iodine (usually via a small pill encased in an impressively large and heavy lead container). Although the pill looks ordinary, it's so radioactive that you'll be told to avoid living things—people and pets—for 48 hours after taking it. You'll also be told to suck on sour candies, which will prevent the radiation from doing damage to your salivary glands. (Don't spit on anything, though, as your saliva—and, for that matter, your clothes—will be radioactive for the next 30 days.)

The iodine from the pill will be ignored by the rest of your body and travel straight to your throat, where it'll be eagerly absorbed by whatever thyroid cells remain. If you have papillary or follicular cancer, its cells absorb the iodine—and the radiation will obliterate them. (It'll also kill whatever benign thyroid cells remain; but because your thyroid is now gone, that doesn't matter.)

If all goes well, this treatment will make you cancer-free, eliminating the possibility of stray thyroid cancer cells eventually spreading to other parts of your body. The only downside is the same as that carried by any radiation treatment—long-term, it poses the risk of initiating cancer itself. But in this case, the positive outcome of annihilating currently existing cancer more than makes up for the remote possibility of developing cancer years later from the radiation.

Treatment for Life

If your entire thyroid is removed, you've effectively become hypothyroid. You'll therefore need to take thyroid medication—typically, a pill or two every morning—for the rest of your life.

You can find information about medication options in Chapters 8 and 9. In your case, your first choice should be desiccated thyroid, or a mix of desiccated and synthetic thyroid. Synthetic medications (such as Synthroid and Cytomel) can be fine if your thyroid is still partially functioning. But because you'll be depending entirely on pills for your thyroid hormones, you should choose desiccated thyroid, which is the only medication that will provide your body with not only T4 and T3, but also T2 (which has been found to be significant for metabolism and weight loss) and T1 (which is currently a mystery to science, but could well serve a purpose not yet discovered).

You should also make a point of seeing your doctor every 6–12 months for follow-up visits. That's especially true if you've had radioactive iodine therapy, because there's a special test you can take one year after the treatment to check on whether it's been successful. Meanwhile, feel comforted in knowing the chances are about 97 percent that your treatment worked as planned and you're entirely healthy again.

Julie's Story

If you'd like a down-to-earth example of what going through the diagnostic and treatment process is like, the experience of my patient Julie is typical.

While curling her hair shortly after her 38th birthday, Julie noticed a lump the size of a marble protruding from her neck. She thought it was quite prominent and was surprised she hadn't spotted it before. Then it occurred to Julie that it might have grown quickly. She realized it could be serious and needed to be checked out.

Julie's family doctor saw her the following week. After feeling her throat, he told her it was probably just a swollen lymph node. "These things happen all the time," he said. "Don't worry about it, but come back next month if it's still there."

A week later, Julie's lump had clearly grown larger, so she made another appointment with her doctor. When he examined her neck again, he found the lump was now over 1 centimeter. "I'm sending you to get an ultrasound," he said. "That'll help us know what's going on."

The ultrasound was arranged for the following week. While waiting for it, Julie could think of little else. During her test, Julie tried to get some information from the face of the technician, but he was unreadable. After it was done, she asked him what he thought. "All I can do is take the images," he said. "I'm not qualified to evaluate. But your doctor will receive the results within a few days."

In fact, Julie's doctor called her the next day. "It's not a lymph node," he said. "It's a thyroid nodule. I'm referring you to an ENT."

The next week, Julie was seen by an ear, nose, and throat surgeon. After a manual exam, he conducted a fine needle aspiration biopsy, taking six tiny samples of Julie's nodule with a needle and syringe. Although Julie pressed, the doctor was unwilling to make any guesses about her condition. "I'll probably have the results tomorrow, though," he said. "I'll call you when they come in."

The next day, Julie was unable to concentrate on anything as she waited anxiously for the call. She hoped it would happen in the morning, but it didn't. She stayed by her desk during lunch, just in case. When 4 pm rolled by, Julie stopped waiting and called the doctor's office. "I'm glad you got in touch," the receptionist said. "The doctor had tried to call you, but it looks like two digits of your phone number accidentally got transposed. Let me put you through now." After a moment, Julie was on the line with the ENT.

Julie fastened on the calm tone in his voice and told herself it meant the results came back negative. Then he said, "You tested positive for papillary cancer of the thyroid. However, the cells don't appear to be very aggressive." All Julie really heard at that moment was, "You have cancer."

The following day, Julie met with the ENT, and he calmly assured her that her odds were excellent. "The surgery alone will probably cure you," he said. "But we'll give you a dose of radiation afterward to be extra safe. With your permission, I'll make the arrangements."

Given the schedule of the ENT and the anesthesiologist, plus Julie needing prior authorization from her insurance provider, the operation was scheduled to take place in three weeks. Julie began to feel everyone was taking this far too casually. During those three weeks, she did little other than fixate on the malignant lump she felt was going to end her life.

When the ENT performed the surgery, he found two nodules—the one that had already been noticed, which had since grown to over 2 centimeters, and another nodule that was 1.5 centimeters. They were both on the left lobe. But based on a discussion with Julie before the operation, the ENT removed her entire thyroid so Julie could feel certain the cancer wouldn't spread.

When Julie woke up afterward, the ENT told her the operation was a success. He also told her that she wouldn't be given thyroid hormones for six weeks, "so when you take the radioactive iodine, any remaining cancer cells will suck it up like a vacuum cleaner."

Six weeks later, in a hypothyroid state that had made her thoroughly fatigued and 10 pounds heavier, Julie was given 130 millicuries of radioactive iodine. She stayed away from people and other living things for two days. During this time there was some swelling under her jaw, but sucking on sour candies made it go away.

Afterward Julie made an appointment with an endocrinologist and was overjoyed to finally be allowed to take thyroid medication.

Over the next couple of months, Julie was relieved that the surgery, the radiation, and most importantly the cancer was behind her. However, she noticed clear and continuing symptoms of fatigue; plus her hair started thinning, and she was starting to feel inexplicably depressed. Julie's endocrinologist ordered thyroid blood tests. When the lab results arrived, her doctor told Julie that her thyroid dosage appeared fine, so nothing else needed to be done.

After a few more months, Julie's hair started falling out. No longer trusting her endocrinologist, Julie made an appointment with me; and I found she was still hypothyroid. Her doctor had misinterpreted her lab results and given her too low a dosage. Further, he'd put her on a T4-only medication, which wasn't as appropriate for Julie as a medication that also provides T3 and T2.

I switched Julie to desiccated thyroid and a higher dosage. Within two months, Julie felt entirely healthy again.

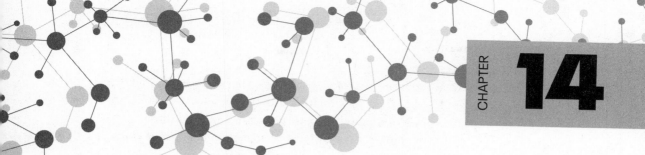

Adrenal Gland Diseases

As explained in Chapter 7, it's possible to be hypothyroid but labeled "normal" on blood tests because the ranges used by most labs are too broad. To make life even more complicated, you can be hypothyroid and labeled "normal" on blood tests because your thyroid really *is* functioning normally. This paradox stems from a pair of endocrine glands called the *adrenal glands* that your thyroid relies on to be effective.

Spotlighting Your Adrenal Glands

The adrenal glands are two small triangle-shaped lumps of tissue residing over your kidneys.

Your adrenals are divided into four sections: an outer *cortex* with three layers, and an inner *medulla*. Each section produces hormones regulating bodily functions vital to your health. These can roughly be summarized as *salt, sugar, sex,* and *stress:*

○ **Salt:** The outermost cortex layer produces hormones such as *aldosterone* that control the amount of sodium and water in your body and regulate your blood pressure.

○ **Sugar:** The middle cortex layer makes the critical hormone *cortisol,* whose many functions include regulating your blood's glucose levels (along with your pancreas), controlling your blood pressure (along with aldosterone), healing inflammations, and enabling your thyroid hormones to enter cells.

○ **Sex:** The innermost cortex layer creates the sex hormones testosterone and estrogen (as a backup for your testicles or ovaries, which produce the same sex hormones).

O **Stress:** The medulla produces *adrenaline,* a hormone that's triggered when you're in a dangerous or unexpected situation. Adrenaline increases your heart rate, expands your blood vessels and air passages, and makes other subtle changes that help you react instantly to whatever trouble comes your way by either battling or running (commonly called *fight or flight*).

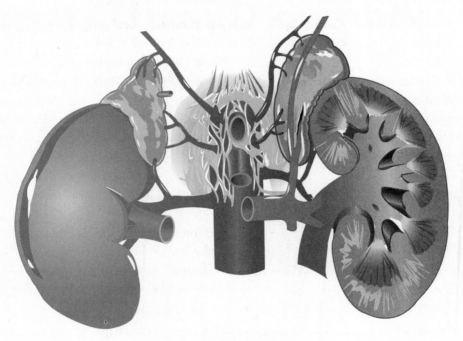

The adrenal glands
(Licensed from Shutterstock Images)

When a Good Thyroid Seems Bad

The adrenal hormone most important to your thyroid is cortisol, which plays two key roles. First, cortisol helps convert the T4 that leaves your thyroid (or that you're taking via medication) into T3. That's a vital function, because T4 is merely a storage state; your body can make use of only T3. In addition, cortisol gives T3 the ability to penetrate a cell's membrane. Once inside a cell, the T3 powers up the cell's mitochondria, providing your body with the energy it needs.

The partnership between your thyroid and your adrenals works beautifully when both glands are healthy. If your adrenal glands start underperforming, however, there won't be enough cortisol to convert T4 into all the T3 you need. Worse, there won't be enough cortisol to allow T3 to penetrate your cells. That means even if your thyroid is doing its job perfectly, your body won't benefit from it because a certain amount of T3 will be blocked from accessing your mitochondria.

Conversely, if your adrenal glands are overperforming, then you'll have too much cortisol in your system, and that's just as much of a problem because excessive cortisol prevents mitochondria from absorbing thyroid hormones. The result is the same—the mitochondria don't get recharged, depriving you of energy vital to your health.

In either case, you'll end up in a hypothyroid state. Your thyroid blood tests will all show up as normal...because your thyroid really *is* healthy and performing its job perfectly. What needs to be diagnosed and treated are your adrenal glands.

Underactive Adrenals

If your adrenal glands are underperforming, you might have *Addison's disease* (also called *adrenal insufficiency*). This refers to a physical problem with your adrenals, such as a genetic defect, or an autoimmune disorder in which your adrenals are being attacked by antibodies. Addison's disease is relatively rare, affecting 1 in 100,000 people.

Alternatively, you might have a problem with your pituitary gland, which controls the activity of your adrenals via a hormone called *ACTH* (also known as *adrenocorticotropic hormone* or *corticotropin*). If for some reason your pituitary starts producing too little ACTH, your adrenal glands—even though perfectly healthy—will underperform because they're following the "orders" conveyed by the ACTH. This is called *secondary adrenal insufficiency*, as the cause is indirect—the problem is really with your pituitary gland, but your adrenals behave as if they're ailing. Further, if this condition is left untreated, over time your adrenals really *will* become damaged, because they'll shrink from lack of use. This condition is much more common than Addison's disease.

Another cause for underperformance is a shortage of the chemical building blocks that fuel hormone production. For example, your adrenals require cholesterol to make cortisol. If your body is having trouble getting cholesterol to your adrenals or if you're taking medication that interferes with cholesterol, your adrenal glands won't have enough raw material to do their job.

As another example, your adrenal glands are secondary suppliers of the sex hormones testosterone and estrogen, essentially backing up the primary production from your testicles or ovaries. At the age when women begin menopause and men's testicles start producing less testosterone (sometimes referred to as *andropause*), the adrenals are required to pick up the slack. If there was a barely adequate amount of chemical ingredients to start with, the increased demand for sex hormones will force the adrenals to cut back on other hormones—including cortisol. For this reason, if you're going to have an adrenal problem, it's most likely to happen at around age 45–55.

Finally, some doctors believe the number one source of adrenal problems is *adrenal fatigue,* or *hypoadrenalism,* which occurs as a three-stage process. When life hands you the occasional hardship, your adrenals will produce extra hormones to help you get through it and will then return to normal. This first stage is called *compensation,* and is perfectly healthy.

If such strains become frequent, though, or if they become exceptionally severe, your adrenals are likely to overreact and produce more hormones than are good for you. This stage is called *overcompensation.*

If the stress then continues over a long period of time, the wear and tear on your adrenals might eventually cause them to lose the ability to produce even normal levels of hormones. This third stage is called *decompensation.*

If this happens to you, your adrenals are likely to *subtly* underperform. The symptoms won't be as severe as those of Addison's disease, but they'll still impair your quality of life. The good news is adrenal fatigue can often be managed with over-the-counter remedies that have virtually no side effects.

Identifying Underactivity

Because your adrenal glands regulate blood sugar, salt, blood pressure, and stress responses, there are some quick and easy things you can do on your own as a first rough check on whether they're underperforming.

First, try delaying or skipping a meal and see if it's any harder to do than usual. If so, that could mean you've become *hypoglycemic*—low on blood sugar—which, in turn, could mean a shortage of cortisol.

Also notice if you have any other symptoms of hypoglycemia, which include frequent hunger (especially for sugar or starch), fatigue, impaired judgment, confusion, nausea, anxiety, and shakiness.

In addition, note whether you've developed strong cravings for salt. That can indicate a shortage of the adrenal hormone aldosterone.

Next, perform a quick check on your blood pressure. It's easy to take your body's management of blood pressure for granted. But when you stand up, there's quite a bit of complex internal orchestration involved to prevent your blood from abruptly dropping from your brain into your feet. When the adrenal hormones cortisol and aldosterone are low, this mechanism isn't as effective, so try lying down for a few minutes and then abruptly rising. If you become dizzy, feel weak, and/or see spots, it's probably because more blood rushed down from your brain than is normal.

If you'd prefer a more formal version of the blood pressure test, tell your doctor that you want her to check your *orthostatic hypotension*. She'll have you lie down, hook you up to a blood pressure machine, and then ask you to stand. If you're healthy, your systolic (top number) blood pressure will go up 5–10 points. But if you're low on adrenal hormones, it'll drop 10–25 points.

Another test you can perform easily on your own is checking your fight-or-flight response, which is regulated by the hormone adrenaline. First, sit in front of a mirror and turn off the light for a minute, which will make your pupils open wide. Then shine a flashlight across (but not directly into) your eyes and watch how your pupils react for the next 30 seconds. Your irises should instantly contract in response to the light increasing and stay contracted. If you're low on adrenaline, however, it's likely that your irises will contract briefly but then expand; or waver back and forth between contracting and expanding.

One other way you can identify underperforming adrenals is paying attention to your skin (and especially your torso's epidermis). A combination of low cortisol and high ACTH can stimulate the cells that control skin pigmentation, resulting in dark, irregularly shaped spots a few inches long—sometimes called "café au lait spots" because they look like spilled coffee.

Testing for Underactivity

If you have reason to suspect an adrenal problem, you should see an endocrinologist for formal testing of your cortisol levels. Unfortunately, this isn't a straightforward procedure because cortisol varies over the course of a day. If you're on a mainstream schedule, your cortisol level will rise in the morning, peaking at around 7 A.M., and then sink to very low levels at night. Therefore, your doctor will probably take two blood tests—one in the morning and the other in the afternoon—noting the time of day for each so that information can be factored in when evaluating the lab results.

If you happen to work at night and sleep during the day, though, your cortisol patterns might be reversed. And if your schedule shifts from day to day, that makes taking just a couple of blood tests even more problematic. To get around this, some doctors will ask you to collect your urine over a 24-hour period. The total is then tested to determine the cortisol level *on average* for the entire day. The downside is there's no information on highs and lows—that is, how much the cortisol varied from one time of day to another. Therefore, this test is most useful as a supplement to the twice-a-day blood test.

Another approach is what's called a *cortisol challenge test*. This involves measuring your cortisol level; giving you a small (typically 25 microgram) dose of ACTH, which is the hormone your pituitary gland makes to stimulate adrenal activity; waiting an hour or two; and then measuring your cortisol level again. If your adrenal glands are healthy, they should have produced at least twice as much cortisol in response to the ACTH. If they didn't, it's a strong indicator they're ailing. This is an excellent way of obtaining precise information about adrenal performance.

This technique is also useful if you have physical symptoms of adrenal under-performance, but your cortisol levels don't appear to be significantly off-kilter on standard blood tests. Even if you have a tolerable cortisol level when you're sitting calmly in a doctor's office, the challenge test will show if your adrenals are inadequate when faced with stress or other demanding situations that call for extra hormone production.

One other available option is *salivary cortisol testing*. This enables you to enjoy a normal day but take a sample of your saliva every 4–6 hours (using a kit supplied by your doctor), marking the time each sample is taken. Adrenal hormones in your saliva are roughly proportional to those in your blood, so the test results allow your doctor to track your cortisol levels throughout the day. The main disadvantage of this method is hormones attach to red blood cells. It's common to have tiny amounts of blood in the saliva; and even if they're too small to see, they can skew results. But your doctor can instruct you on ways to minimize this problem (such as not brushing your teeth the day of the testing).

It's possible to be hypothyroid from thyroid disease alone and from adrenal disease alone. But you shouldn't discount the possibility of having *both* diseases. If your thyroid starts failing, your adrenals might work harder to compensate and eventually become damaged from the strain. If you notice symptoms of both diseases, it might not be your imagination, and you shouldn't hesitate to get tested for both.

Treating Underactivity

The standard treatment for low cortisol levels is cortisol replacement medication. However, this isn't an ideal solution. Your body needs different amounts of cortisol at different hours of the day. In addition, it requires extra cortisol when you're faced with challenging situations, such as stress or an infection. Taking a pill once a day is a poor substitute for the flexibility and adaptability provided by your adrenal glands.

Further, consuming external cortisol can create new health problems. Cortisol is an anti-inflammatory, so it will stop inflammation wherever it ends up in your body. Because inflammation is an important tool your body uses to repair itself, prolonged use of cortisol replacement risks erosion of your intestinal lining and esophagus.

If your adrenal glands are severely damaged—for example, if you have advanced Addison's disease—then taking cortisol pills for life might be your only realistic option. If you have a choice, though, it's better to first try making your adrenals stronger and more efficient.

Finally, you can make lifestyle changes that ease the strain on your adrenals, such as eating healthy, cutting down on stress, and eliminating toxins. For details, see Chapters 18 and 20.

Overactive Adrenals

As bad as it is to have too little cortisol, it's even worse to have too much of it. The latter condition is called *Cushing's syndrome*, or *hypercortisolism*. Cushing's syndrome often results from cortisol-based medication such as prednisone. Because of its anti-inflammatory properties, cortisol is used to treat such illnesses as asthma, rheumatoid arthritis, lupus, and ulcerative colitis. That's normally fine. But if you take high doses of cortisol for a prolonged period, it will start to break down your tissues, and might do damage to your heart and bones. If this occurs, you can simply taper off your current medication and then switch to one that's not cortisol-based.

More serious is when your adrenal glands are overproducing cortisol. This is relatively rare, occurring most often in adults aged 20–50. It also happens in women in the last trimester of pregnancy because that's a period of substantial hormone changes. Causes include autoimmune disease, in which antibodies attack your adrenals and cause them to enlarge.

Alternatively, your adrenal glands' cells can spawn tumors called *pheochromocytoma*— growing either on the glands or outside of them—that produce hormones independently. The combination of hormones from both your adrenals and the tumors will put you beyond healthy limits.

A more indirect cause that ends up creating the same effect is your body having too much ACTH. This can happen if you're taking medication that contains a high amount of ACTH. It can also result from *adenomas* (non-cancerous tumors) that start growing on your pituitary gland and increase ACTH output. In either case, the extra ACTH forces your adrenals to produce more cortisol than is good for you.

The pituitary gland isn't the only source of ACTH. Extra ACTH can also stem from cancerous tumors—for example, in the lungs or intestines. When this occurs, the symptoms of Cushing's syndrome are a blessing because they'll tip off an astute doctor to the existence of cancers that must be located and destroyed.

Another source of danger is steering your adrenals into developing bad habits. For example, if you're an athlete who trains hard, you're forcing your adrenal glands to produce a lot of extra cortisol. That's usually not a problem if you take care to include adequate periods in between sessions for your body to rest, recover, and reset. But if you're overtraining day after day, your adrenal glands can become so used to over-generating cortisol that they get stuck at that higher setting and will continue to overproduce even if you stop exercising.

Identifying Overactivity

The primary symptom of Cushing's syndrome is gaining a lot of weight, especially in the middle and upper body. Fat is prone to gather around the neck and back (between the shoulder blades). In children, the obesity is accompanied by a slowed rate of growth.

Also, there's often facial swelling that creates a rounded "moon face" and loss of lean body mass resulting in relatively thin arms and legs.

Further, too much cortisol thins the skin, making it easy for mere bumps to bruise or tear skin. The fragility of the skin, coupled with the weight gain, can also result in pink or purple stretch marks on the torso, arms, buttocks, thighs, legs, and/or breasts. Thinning, brittle hair and hair loss is common as well.

Because cortisol reduces immune responses, wounds may happen more often and take an extra-long time to heal. You could also start developing aches and pains in your hips, shoulders, and lower back. And you might be the first to catch any illness going around and among the last to recover.

If your adrenals produce excess adrenaline, your emotions can become heightened and intensify your emotions, making you feel anxious, euphoric, depressed, or even psychotic.

If you're a woman and your adrenals overproduce sex hormones, this can cause your menstrual cycles to become irregular, or to stop altogether. Further, you might get unusual patterns of hair growth and facial acne. And if you're a man, the overdose of cortisol can reduce your sex drive and impair erections.

Additional symptoms include high blood sugar, increased thirst and urination, fatigue, weakness, and hypertension.

Cushing's syndrome must be taken seriously. If left untreated for a long time, it can lead to diabetes, osteoporosis, heart disease, and death.

Testing for Overactivity

Your doctor typically will check for adrenal overproduction by giving you v1 milligram of dexamethasone, which is a powerful synthetic version of cortisol, and then testing your blood's cortisol levels both the same day and the next day. If you're healthy, your pituitary gland should pick up on the fact your body has more cortisol than it needs and lower its production of ACTH. If the following day's blood test doesn't show reduced cortisol, then your pituitary gland has a problem. In this case, some other part of your body (typically, a tumor) is generating ACTH on its own; or your adrenals aren't responding normally to the ACTH.

Alternatively, your doctor can test cortisol levels by having you collect either your urine or your saliva over a 24-hour period. If she determines there's a problem, she'll order a CT scan of your adrenals and MRI of your pituitary gland to look for anything out of the ordinary, such as growths on the glands.

Treating Overactivity

There are some drugs that either lower the body's production of cortisol or lower the effects of cortisol, such as ketoconazole and metyrapone. However, their effectiveness is limited.

Therefore, the most common solution is surgery. For example, if an adenoma is found on the pituitary gland, the growth will be cut out. If the surgery restores your glands to health, then nothing more needs to be done.

However, if the surgery either removed or damaged your pituitary or adrenal glands, you'll need to deal with a shortage of cortisol (as described earlier in this chapter).

For more information about adrenal issues—and also other diseases that frequently accompany thyroid disease—see Chapter 21, "Secondary Problems."

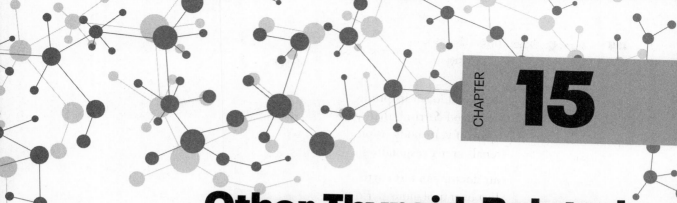

CHAPTER 15

Other Thyroid-Related Diseases

So far, this book has covered hypothyroidism, hyperthyroidism, and cancer. These diseases cause more than 95 percent of all thyroid-related problems. However, they aren't the whole story.

Hundreds of thousands of people are diagnosed every year with other thyroid-related illnesses, including parathyroid disease, thyroiditis (inflamed thyroid), thyroid eye disease, and multiple endocrine neoplasia (thyroid tumors).

If you have reason to believe you're suffering from one of these less common conditions, this chapter will provide the information you need for seeking an accurate diagnosis and successful treatment.

Parathyroid Disease

Directly behind your thyroid are small glands, each about the size of a grain of rice, called *parathyroid glands*. There are typically four of them, but the number can vary from person to person.

The Parathyroids

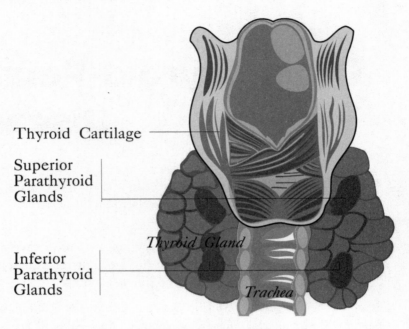

Thyroid Cartilage

Superior
Parathyroid
Glands

Thyroid Gland

Inferior
Parathyroid
Glands

Trachea

The parathyroid glands
(Licensed from Shutterstock Images)

While your parathyroid glands reside behind your thyroid, they have an entirely separate function: secreting *parathyroid hormone* (*PTH*; also called parathormone or parathyrin), which moves calcium out of your bones and into your bloodstream.

PTH works in opposition with a thyroid hormone called *calcitonin*, which moves calcium out of your blood and into your bones. One of the reasons that overdosing on thyroid medication can damage your bones is that it hinders your thyroid from releasing calcitonin.

How much calcium you have in your body ultimately depends on how much you consume, but PTH and calcitonin adjust how much goes in the blood and how much goes elsewhere.

That might not sound like a big deal. However, calcium affects such vital functions as preventing your bones from breaking down and transmitting signals to your muscles, which among other things, ensures that your heart keeps beating.

Maintaining your calcium levels within the narrow range your body requires (from 8.5 to 10.2 milligrams per deciliter of blood) is a delicate task, so anything that throws your parathyroid glands off-kilter can result in serious consequences.

Experts estimate roughly 100,000 Americans a year develop parathyroid disease. It's about three times more likely to occur in women, and is most common after age 50.

Parathyroid disease can result in abnormal calcium levels and ongoing symptoms such as fatigue, confusion, depression, muscle pain, osteoporosis, and kidney stones. If left unchecked, it can also increase your risk for strokes and heart attacks. It's therefore important to detect and treat this disease as soon as possible.

Detecting Parathyroid Disease

Parathyroid disease usually can be detected—or ruled out—with some simple blood tests.

Specifically, your doctor needs to take a small amount of your blood and then order a group of lab tests called a *comprehensive metabolic panel* (also known as a CMP, Chemistry Panel, Chemistry Screen, or SMAC Test). These tests are so standard that many doctors perform them on their patients routinely as part of an annual checkup. They identify the levels of a variety of critical chemicals in your bloodstream...including calcium.

If your blood's calcium level is either too high or too low, there's something wrong. The issue could be parathyroid disease, or it could be something even more serious such as cancer. Your doctor should therefore conduct follow-up blood tests—including one that measures PTH—to home in on the cause.

If your doctor fails to identify the reason for your abnormal serum calcium and says, "Don't worry about it, it's probably nothing," you should find another doctor who'll do the job right. Because possible causes range from parathyroid problems that can rob years from your life if left untreated to even deadlier diseases such as cancer, a discovery of a calcium level that's off-kilter should never be ignored.

You should also be aware that even if your serum calcium test results come back as normal, that doesn't necessarily mean you don't have parathyroid disease. This more complex situation will be explained shortly.

There are several varieties of parathyroid disease, which are covered next.

Hyperparathyroidism

If your parathyroid glands secrete too much PTH (the hormone that moves calcium from your bones to your bloodstream), ignoring signals that the ideal calcium level in your blood has already been achieved, you have *hyperparathyroidism.* This disease has three main types: primary, secondary, and parathyroid cancer.

If you have primary hyperparathyroidism, a benign tumor (adenoma) has grown on a parathyroid gland and is producing too much PTH. In more than 80 percent of cases, it's a single parathyroid gland that's overactive. But sometimes two, three, or all the parathyroid glands have these tumors.

Overdoing the transfer of calcium from your bones to your blood might not sound like a big deal, but it can lead to any of the following issues:

- Fatigue
- Irritability
- Impaired sleep
- Confusion and/or memory loss
- Depression and/or anxiety
- Nausea and/or vomiting
- Constipation
- Muscle pain
- Bone loss
- Bone fractures
- Osteoporosis
- Gastric ulcers

O Pancreatitis

O Kidney stones

O Kidney failure

O Breast cancer

O Stroke

O Heart attack

This condition can typically be treated with minimally invasive surgery to remove the tumorous gland(s). If you have to go this route, seek the most experienced parathyroid surgeon available (see the next section). In most cases, your remaining parathyroid glands will pick up the slack—that is, produce just enough additional hormones to make up for the gland(s) removed.

Most primary hyperparathyroidism symptoms occur so slowly and subtly that you aren't even aware you have them. After your surgery, though, you'll probably notice improvements that make you realize you'd been operating at less than 100 percent in a variety of areas.

If you have secondary hyperparathyroidism, your parathyroids are working harder than usual to produce PTH, but for a good reason: your body doesn't have enough calcium. The most common reason for this is kidney failure. However, it can also occur if you aren't consuming enough calcium, your digestive system isn't absorbing calcium efficiently, or your body isn't making enough vitamin D (typically because you're not spending enough time in sunlight). Dealing with the cause of the calcium shortage will end the secondary hyperparathyroidism.

Finally, less than 1 percent of hyperparathyroid cases are parathyroid cancer. This occurs when a parathyroid gland develops a malignant overgrowth of cells that then wildly overproduce PTH. This condition is treated with surgery to remove the cancerous parathyroid gland. Again, seek the most experienced parathyroid surgeon available (see directly below). After the operation, your remaining parathyroid glands will typically secrete enough hormones to make up for the removed gland.

Hypoparathyroidism

If your parathyroid glands produce too little PTH—in other words, fail to move sufficient calcium from your bones to maintain a normal level of calcium in your bloodstream—you have a disease called *hypoparathyroidism*.

Ironically, the major cause of hypoparathyroidism is treatment for thyroid disease. If a surgeon needs to remove part or all of your thyroid—which is usually the first step in treatment for thyroid cancer (see Chapter 13), and occasionally for hyperthyroidism (see Chapter 12)—there's a risk the surgeon will accidentally damage one or more of your parathyroid glands, which reside behind it. This is one of the scenarios doctors worry about most when considering thyroid surgery...especially because the precise number, location, and size of parathyroids can be quite different from patient to patient.

Similarly, radiation (in the form of radioiodine ablation, as described in Chapters 12 and 13) can be used to either destroy a thyroid's cancer cells or reduce the thyroid's mass to treat hyperthyroidism. Even though the parathyroids aren't being targeted by the radioiodine, there's a risk they'll become damaged simply because of how close they are to the radioactive thyroid cells. In addition, the radiation exposure poses a long-term risk of the parathyroids developing cancer or other growths themselves.

If you ever require a thyroid or parathyroid operation, the best way to avoid these scenarios is to seek the most experienced thyroid or parathyroid surgeon available.

Hypoparathyroidism can also spontaneously occur in someone who's never had neck surgery. This is rare, and no one knows why it happens.

One other way hypoparathyroidism can develop is if your body lacks enough magnesium. This is easily solved by consuming foods rich in magnesium, such as kale, broccoli, figs, bananas, nuts and seeds, and legumes; and by cutting out alcohol, which lowers magnesium levels.

Symptoms of hypoparathyroidism can include:

○ Tingling in the hands and fingers, in the toes, or around the mouth

○ Muscle aches or cramps

○ Twitching or spasms

○ Fatigue

○ Painful menstrual periods

○ Depression and/or anxiety

In most cases, your doctor will treat your hypoparathyroidism by having you take calcium supplements several times a day along with a high dose of vitamin D once a day.

Interpreting Complex Test Results

As explained previously, if a blood test shows your calcium level is either too high or too low, any good doctor will investigate via further tests.

Complicating matters is that in around 20 percent of cases, a calcium level will test within the normal range even though the patient has parathyroid disease. So if at least several of your symptoms match the ones described in this chapter, insist on your doctor giving you calcium *and* PTH blood tests. This is a condition you want to catch early, rather than wait until you develop clearer symptoms, such as distinct patterns of bone loss or kidney stones.

Once your doctor receives the results of your calcium and PTH blood tests, listen carefully to his evaluation and ask for a copy of what the lab sent him. You can then double-check your doctor's interpretation of the lab numbers against the chart below. If they don't match up, discuss it with your doctor and be open to seeking a second opinion.

		Calcium (8.5–10.4 mg/dL)			
		Low	Normal	High normal	Elevated
PTH (10–65 nmol/L)	Low	Hypoparathyroidism	Hypoparathyroidism	High calcium due to excessive intake or malignancy	High calcium due to excessive intake or malignancy
	Normal	Hypoparathyroidism	Healthy	Primary Hyperparathyroidism	Primary Hyperparathyroidism
	Elevated	Secondary Hyperparathyroidism (low calcium due to low intake, chronic kidney disease, etc.)	Primary Hyperparathyroidism	Primary Hyperparathyroidism	Primary Hyperparathyroidism

Thyroiditis

If your thyroid feels swollen and inflamed, you might have *thyroiditis*, which typically stems from Hashimoto's disease (see Chapter 5). However, certain varieties of thyroiditis are (usually) temporary illnesses. They include painful subacute thyroiditis, silent thyroiditis, postpartum thyroiditis, and iodine-induced thyroiditis.

Painful Subacute Thyroiditis

Painful subacute thyroiditis (also known as *de Quervain's thyroiditis* or *subacute granulomatous thyroiditis*) typically occurs after a respiratory infection—for example, after you've had the mumps, the flu, or some other virus. If your body's attacks on the virus create high inflammation, that can, in turn, spawn antibodies that end up attacking your thyroid. If this occurs, you'll probably feel neck pain. If your thyroid swells, you might also have some trouble swallowing or talking, and/or become feverish and weak.

In addition, because nerves can sometimes carry signals of distress beyond the area causing the problem, you might feel pain in your ears, jaw, and/or face.

Further, you'll become hyperthyroid, which means—among other things—that your heart might start beating too rapidly.

Your doctor can diagnose this condition by giving you an *iodine uptake and thyroid scan*. This involves injecting you with or having you swallow a tiny amount of radioactive iodine, waiting 6–24 hours, and then scanning your neck to get a clear picture of what's going on in your thyroid.

If you have this condition, your doctor should give you a nonsteroidal anti-inflammatory drug—essentially, a prescription-strength equivalent of ibuprofen—to reduce the inflammation. (If that doesn't work, she can alternatively prescribe corticosteroids, which are steroid-based anti-inflammatory drugs.) In addition, your doctor should prescribe beta blockers to prevent your heart from beating too quickly.

With the help of these medications, the chances are good that you'll be okay until the condition clears itself up. However, in rare cases—and especially if the illness is left untreated—the disease can so stress the thyroid that a permanent condition of hypothyroidism results.

Silent Thyroiditis

Silent thyroiditis (also known as *painless thyroiditis* or *subacute lymphocytic thyroiditis*) is another condition in which your body turns on itself by creating antibodies that attack your thyroid.

Unlike painful subacute thyroiditis, this illness isn't spawned by a viral infection; no one knows what causes it. And while it enlarges your thyroid, it doesn't make the thyroid tender and prone to pain.

As with painful subacute thyroiditis, your doctor can diagnose this condition by giving you an iodine uptake and thyroid scan.

If you have silent thyroiditis, you'll start out as hyperthyroid. During this period, your doctor might prescribe beta blockers to prevent your heart from beating too quickly. The hyperthyroidism will typically last for 2–3 months. You might then become hypothyroid for 2–3 months and require thyroid medication (see Chapter 8). After this phase, your body will probably cure itself, leaving you healthy. In rare cases, though, the thyroid can become so stressed by the illness that it ends up remaining in the hypothyroid state.

Postpartum Thyroiditis

If you're pregnant, your body will make changes to your immune system during and after the pregnancy to ensure the health of both you and your baby. These changes are normally harmless, but 5–7 percent of women spawn antibodies that end up attacking the thyroid. (Most at risk are women with type 1 diabetes.) This typically happens 2–6 months after the baby is born, but it can also occur up to a year later.

Postpartum thyroiditis might also occur following a miscarriage or an elective abortion, which puts the body through the same kind of immune system changes.

The symptoms, diagnosis, and treatment for postpartum thyroiditis are the same as those for silent thyroiditis. With time and patience, this illness usually rides itself out. For about 20 percent of women, however, the thyroid ends up remaining in a hypothyroid state. And for the other 80 percent, this illness is likely to recur with subsequent pregnancies and/or as a result of the hormonal changes that come with the onset of menopause.

Iodine-Induced Thyroiditis

For your thyroid to function properly, you need to consume 50–199 micrograms (mcg) of iodine per day.

If you overdose on iodine, however, you might get *iodine-induced thyroiditis.* Overdosing can result from taking an over-the-counter thyroid product containing an iodine megadose, or by regularly eating a lot of seafood or other iodine-rich food. It can also occur if you were on a low-iodine diet for a long time and then abruptly switched to a normal intake of iodine, shocking your thyroid into processing more iodine than it's used to.

The problem is that as much as 45 percent of people are estimated to have latent thyroid disease—that is, antibodies floating around for Hashimoto's disease or Graves' disease that normally don't do any harm. But when your thyroid is disrupted by an abrupt change in iodine or by steady iodine megadoses, this can trigger the antibodies into actively attacking your thyroid. As a result, you'll suddenly become hypothyroid or hyperthyroid.

The simple solution is to stop taking the excess iodine. In many cases, your body will heal and you'll become healthy again. However, it's possible that once the thyroid disease is triggered, it becomes permanent. If this happens, you'll need to be treated for either hypothyroidism (see Chapter 8) or hyperthyroidism (see Chapter 12).

For suggestions on how to reduce your daily iodine intake, see Chapter 18.

Thyroid Eye Disease

If you have Graves' disease—or, more rarely, Hashimoto's disease—there's a chance the same type of antibodies attacking your thyroid will enlarge your eye cells and ocular tissues.

Symptoms you might feel in your eyes include:

○ Continual pain, or pain when looking around

○ Dryness or itchiness

○ Double vision or other impaired vision

○ Bloodshot eyes

○ Inflammation and swelling

○ Swelling in the orbital tissues that can cause your eyeball to push forward, creating a wide-eyed, bulging look

The usual treatments are eye drops and ointments to ease suffering until the disease goes away.

Thyroid eye disease can subside for a while and then return. If it disappears for more than six months, it's usually gone for good. For about 3 percent of patients who have thyroid eye disease, however, the disease won't end by itself. In these cases, surgery is required.

Also, even if the disease disappears on its own, the wide-eyed look can sometimes remain. When this happens, surgery is required to restore the eyes to normal.

MEN Syndrome

Roughly 1 in 30,000 people has a genetic defect called *multiple endocrine neoplasia 1* (*MEN1*), which is also known as *Werner's syndrome*; or *multiple endocrine neoplasia 2* (*MEN2*), which is also known as *Sipple's syndrome*.

MEN1 causes various endocrine glands—the thyroid, parathyroids, pancreas, pituitary, and/or adrenals—to start growing tumors at the same time. These tumors usually aren't cancerous, but the enlargement of the glands leads to an overproduction of hormones. This can show up as a wide variety of symptoms—headaches, blurred vision, racing heartbeat, and scores of other possibilities—because these glands affect almost every area of your body. Left untreated, the excess hormones can severely damage your quality of life and even take years off your life.

MEN1 runs in families, and it can be detected through gene testing. It can also be diagnosed through blood tests that check hormone levels. There's currently no cure for MEN1. However, once detected, the tumors it creates can be removed via surgery, or the excess hormones can be suppressed via medication.

MEN2 is like MEN1 in that it causes endocrine glands to grow tumors. Unfortunately, with MEN2 the tumors are usually cancerous. That means they can spread from the glands to other parts of your body, which makes them deadly.

MEN2 also runs in families and can be detected through gene testing. If you're unlucky enough to win this genetic lottery, you should be closely monitored. If or when cancerous tumors occur, they can be destroyed using surgery and/or radiation.

It's tough enough to deal with one of the thyroid conditions in this chapter. But it's even worse if you're also afflicted by a secondary disease, such as diabetes or an adrenal disorder, and your doctor doesn't realize it because he's focused on your thyroid. To fully recover your health, it's important to identify and treat *all* relevant issues. If you suspect your symptoms go beyond your thyroid, read Chapter 21, "Secondary Problems."

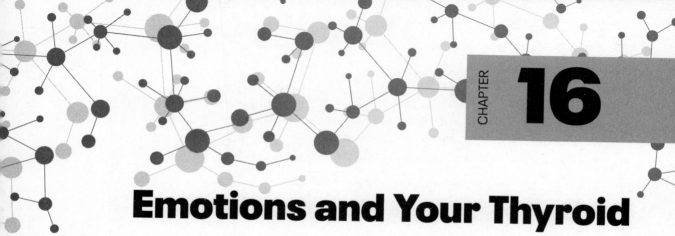

CHAPTER 16

Emotions and Your Thyroid

One of the worst aspects of thyroid disease is the havoc it can play with our minds and emotions. The physical symptoms of a thyroid problem, such as gaining weight or losing hair, are easy to spot. Mental symptoms such as clinical depression or anxiety are more subtle...and more likely to be dismissed as being the result of stress, personal issues, or "just your imagination."

However, they're very real illnesses. Millions of people struggle with mental disorders, and many of them could be cured if they realized the source of their pain was an easily treatable thyroid condition.

How Hormones Rule Us

The relationship between our intangible minds and physical bodies has been a topic of conjecture and wonder for ages. While no one understands all the nuances of the mind-body connection, it's undeniable that your thoughts and moods are heavily influenced by the "chemical soup" that's constantly circulating in your blood and interacting with your brain. And among the chemicals that have the biggest impact are hormones.

If you're a woman, you know how enormously moods can be affected by the hormonal upheavals that accompany PMS, menstruation, pregnancy, post-pregnancy, and menopause.

And if you're a man, think back to when you became an adolescent, your thoughts suddenly started focusing on sex, and you became more aggressive. Also recall that as you grew older, your sex drive became less urgent and your attitude mellowed. These changes were orchestrated by your hormones.

More specifically, each cell in your body has multiple mini-programs built in called *receptors*. When a hormone designed to generate an activity enters a cell containing a receptor for that activity, the hormone behaves like the ignition key in an engine and turns on the receptor. The cell then performs the appropriate action.

When it comes to thyroid hormones, the activities that can be activated include energy production, cell growth, and the manufacturing of critical chemicals. That might not sound significant within the context of one tiny cell, but your brain is composed of *billions* of cells. When hormones activate many receptors in your brain at the same time, the emotional effects can be overwhelming.

Unfortunately, the same holds true when brain cells that would normally be activated suddenly aren't—for example, due to a hormone shortage caused by hypothyroidism. The painful numbness of this lack of activity has been described by some depressed patients as "the void."

> Everything was black. The trees were black, the road was black. You can't believe how the colors change unless you have it. There's just no color. It's scary.
>
> —Pulitzer Prize winning humorist, and depression survivor, Art Buchwald

Many people feel embarrassed or ashamed about having a disease that impacts their emotions. In the past, there's been a terrible lack of understanding about such illnesses, and a tendency to blame those who have them. Given what medical science now knows about these problems, however, there should be no more of a stigma associated with depression or anxiety than there is with having asthma or diabetes. All these conditions are the result of something gone wrong with the body's internal chemistry—and they're all treatable.

Diagnosing and Treating Depression

> What's really diabolical about it is that if there were a pill over there, 10 feet from me, that you could guarantee would lift me out of it, it would be too much trouble to go get it.
>
> —Emmy winning TV host and author Dick Cavett, speaking about his depression

If you're hypothyroid, one of the results of your brain having an insufficient amount of T3 can be clinical depression. While the cause is straightforward—your brain isn't being supplied with the energy it needs—the consequences can be devastating. As many who've suffered this illness will attest, almost nothing compares to its special kind of pain.

People who've never experienced clinical depression often mistake it for no more than sadness, and their response might be to tell you to "get over it" or "cheer up." That's like suggesting to someone with cancer to "just tell your cells to be healthy again." A more pragmatic approach is needed.

The good news is if your depression stems entirely from a lack of thyroid hormones, taking thyroid medication should soon cure it. This is often so effective that it can seem like magic. However, the medication is simply providing your brain with the chemicals it needs to function properly.

One qualification is that taking T4 alone—for example, in the form of Synthroid—might not be effective. No one is sure why, but when it comes to depression, taking T3 directly (as opposed to relying on your body to convert T4 to T3) typically works best. Therefore, taking any of the following is likely to work:

○ Desiccated thyroid (such as Nature-Throid), which is a natural mix of T4 and T3.

○ A mix of Synthroid (synthetic T4) and Cytomel (synthetic T3).

○ A mix of desiccated thyroid and Synthroid. This can make sense when you need a T4-to-T3 ratio that can't be achieved with desiccated thyroid alone (see Chapter 9).

If your only problem was an underperforming thyroid, then once you're on the right hormone dosage—and especially the right amount of direct T3—your depression should disappear. If your depression lifts to a degree but doesn't go away, then there could be causes for it beyond your thyroid. In this case, you should keep taking T3, but also pursue other treatments, such as the suggestions in Chapter 18, exercise, talk therapy, and/or antidepressant medication.

Diagnosing and Treating Anxiety

Anxiety is the rust of life, destroying its brightness and weakening its power.

—Anonymous

Anxiety is a frequent symptom of hyperthyroidism. As your metabolism speeds up, you're likely to become more tense, nervous, and apprehensive about everyday events for no apparent reason. In addition, your heart might beat exceptionally fast, making you feel as if you drank a pot of coffee.

Victims of anxiety often blame their feelings on stress. But it's wise to get tested for a physical cause, including an overactive thyroid, if you weren't anxious previously and nothing notable has changed in your life.

Paradoxically, anxiety can also stem from Hashimoto's disease, which is the primary cause of *hypo*thyroidism.

That's because Hashimoto's breaks down the colloid cells that make up your thyroid. The destruction of these cells progressively shrinks your thyroid until it's unable to produce the amount of hormones you need. However, during the early stages of Hashimoto's, every time a bunch of colloid cells rupture, they release the thyroid hormones they were storing.

This abrupt spurt of extra hormones into your body can make you temporarily hyperthyroid—which might result in feelings of anxiousness, nervousness, and/or irritability. Over time, you'll feel a gradual decline in hormones as your body returns to normal, and as your thyroid works at reduced capacity. But then the Hashimoto's will strike again, and you'll undergo another episode of hyperthyroidism.

This cycle of highs and lows—which is called *Hashitoxicosis*—is likely to create wild mood swings. However, lab test results for your TSH, free T4, and free T3 levels might all show up as normal, because the highs and lows often end up balancing each other out. Unless your doctor happens to take your blood during a period when the Hashimoto's is attacking and your thyroid levels are spiking, standard blood tests might label your thyroid as functioning perfectly.

To account for this, your first blood workup should also cover antibodies. Because Hashimoto's is an autoimmune disease, it's highly likely to be detected via tests for antibodies attacking your thyroid.

It's a good idea to check for antibodies in *any* initial thyroid blood testing. Nonetheless, most doctors neglect this step. So if you're experiencing mood swings, insist that antibody testing be included in your doctor's orders to the lab.

You should also be aware that, in rare cases, antibodies might not turn up in a lab test even though your thyroid is being attacked. So if you still suspect a thyroid issue, don't hesitate to ask for an ultrasound, which will allow your doctor to find physical evidence of damage to your thyroid.

If it turns out your anxiety is being caused by standard hyperthyroidism—for example, the autoimmune disorder Graves' disease—see Chapter 12 for treatment options.

If the cause is Hashitoxicosis, however, then your doctor will prescribe anti-anxiety medication to allow you to "ride out" the periodic attacks. We recommend that you also try the suggestions in Chapter 18, "Reversing Thyroid Disease Through Diet," to see if they help. Otherwise, the Hashimoto's will stabilize over time, putting you into a permanent hypothyroid state that can be managed easily with thyroid pills (see Chapters 8 and 9).

No one knows why, but anxiety can also be a symptom of standard hypothyroidism. This isn't as common as anxiety stemming from an overactive thyroid, but it happens. If you're diagnosed as having low thyroid activity and you feel anxiety, it's not your imagination, and the problem will probably go away once you're on thyroid medication.

Other Mental Disorders

Thyroid symptoms can resemble a wide range of mental problems beyond depression and anxiety. For example, if you're hypothyroid, you might become foggy and confused and have memory lapses that resemble Alzheimer's disease (such as forgetting if it's summer or winter). But while Alzheimer's is incurable and fatal, hypothyroidism can be readily managed with medication.

Doctors who don't recognize thyroid disease are especially a problem for the elderly. An estimated 25 percent of people 75 and older are hypothyroid, but their thyroid-related symptoms will often be misdiagnosed as age-related dementia and go untreated.

As another example, if you're severely hyperthyroid, you might experience hallucinations, delusions, and other symptoms associated with psychosis. Patients are periodically misdiagnosed as suffering from schizophrenia when they simply have an overactive thyroid.

Then again, hyperthyroidism might lead you to become manic—for example, impulsive, reckless, or promiscuous, and skipping sleep for days on end until your body gives out and you "crash." If the hormone spike is due to a Hashimoto's attack, then soon afterward you're likely to swing down the other direction into depression. This high/low cycle can easily be mistaken for bipolar disorder.

A particularly insidious complication with bipolar disorder is that many of the medications used to treat it—especially newer ones such as carbamazepine and Depakote—have side effects that include weight gain, depression, dry skin, hair loss... in other words, signs of hypothyroidism. So if your onset of Hashimoto's is mistaken for bipolar disorder, and you go on to develop full-blown hypothyroidism, it'll be almost impossible to tell from your symptoms. Your doctor will just assume you're experiencing the side effects of the bipolar drugs. There are patients who needlessly suffered for years for just this reason.

Considering that thyroid disease symptoms can so closely mimic both those of mental illnesses and the side effects of medications used to treat them, a wise precaution when seeing a doctor for the first time about a mental issue is to insist on having thyroid blood tests done—including antibody tests. You might find that your problems are stemming entirely from your thyroid.

Alternatively, you might really have the mental illness your symptoms indicate—but *also* have a thyroid problem that's making it *even worse*. For example, if you're bipolar and in addition have even a slight leaning toward hypothyroidism, the latter might make you resistant to the mood stabilizers used to treat bipolar disorders. Doctors who understand this will put you on thyroid medication and adjust the dosage until your T4 and T3 levels are as perfect as possible. (This is analogous to adding T3 to antidepressants. Even if your lab tests show your thyroid to be normal, the added hormones can make your medication more effective.)

One other nasty complication with bipolar disease is that one of its treatments, lithium, is chemically close enough to iodine to be eagerly absorbed by your thyroid. Over time, there's a greater than 30 percent chance this will damage your thyroid and lead to hypothyroidism. Because of this, lithium is seldom the first choice for treating bipolar disorder. For some people, however, lithium works better than anything else. If that applies to you, have your doctor check your thyroid every 2–3 months to make sure it's remaining healthy despite the risk posed by the medication.

Other conditions that can cause emotional upheavals include PMS, perimenopause, and menopause. They're covered next in Chapter 17, "For Women Only."

17

For Women Only

If you're a woman, you're more than five times as likely to develop thyroid disease as a man. Your chances of being struck by a thyroid disorder at some point in your life are as high as 20 percent.

You also have special challenges that men don't. For example, going through hormonal upheavals such as PMS, perimenopause, and menopause isn't fun, even under normal circumstances; but having thyroid disease will make such tough times substantially worse. And if you're having trouble getting pregnant, you should be aware that hypothyroidism might be the cause.

This chapter covers the special impact thyroid disease has on women. In most cases, treatment is quick and easy—if you're empowered with the knowledge of how to recognize a thyroid-related problem and manage it.

PMS

If you have premenstrual syndrome, you're far from alone. PMS has been estimated to affect over 85 percent of women between the ages of 20 and 40. While PMS symptoms are no picnic even when you're healthy, they can magnify when combined with thyroid issues.

To appreciate why, you first need to understand what's happening in your body during your monthly cycle. After you comprehend the causes of PMS and how they interact with thyroid symptoms, you might find that thyroid medication coupled with simple over-the-counter remedies help enormously.

Understanding PMS

If you're typical, your period lasts 3–5 days. If we count the first day of bleeding as day 1, then ovulation occurs on days 10–15, and your whole cycle lasts 28–30 days.

Your ovaries produce two primary hormones, *estrogen* and *progesterone*. They'll begin secreting estrogen a day or two before ovulation. After that your estrogen level will go down for a while, and then reach its highest levels during days 17–23. Progesterone isn't made during the first half of the cycle, but is secreted right after ovulation, then maintained at high levels during days 16–25. That means both estrogen and progesterone are operating in force during days 17–23, with their peak around day 21.

These hormones travel through your entire body, first targeting your brain, your breasts, and your uterus. They next recirculate and go to your liver, where they get bound up by carrier proteins (mostly *glucuronic acid*) and are sent through the bile into your colon. If all goes well, these hormones then leave your body via the stool.

But what often happens during peak hormone production—around day 21—is a certain amount of hormones escape the liver or become loosened from its carrier proteins in the colon, and reenter your bloodstream. They'll then circulate around your body again. As they do, byproducts from these "used" hormones have negative effects on your brain's chemistry.

For example, they can make you feel depressed, anxious, angry, or edgy; make you foggy and forgetful; and lead to mood swings and crying spells. They can also make you crave sugar and/or salt.

The byproducts can additionally affect your breasts, making them enlarged and tender. And they can thicken the uterine lining, making it harder to push out through the cervix, which leads to menstrual pain and cramps.

These hormones with bad byproducts will then return to your liver and colon, but they might escape and recirculate one or two more times before finally exiting your body. The problems they cause are a large reason why you feel uncomfortable a week or so before your period.

Another factor is that the hormones moving through the colon change the colon's chemistry. This can cause nausea, upset stomach, gas, bloating, irregularity, constipa-tion, and/or diarrhea. The high level of hormones can also raise the background level of inflammation in your body, leading to backaches, headaches, and joint and muscle pain.

On top of all that, estrogen blocks T3 from entering your cells' membranes. This means when you have more estrogen in your system, fewer cells in your body can make use of available thyroid hormones.

If your thyroid is working normally, you'll simply ride out the third week in your cycle when estrogen is peaking and keeping you from receiving the full benefit of available T3. But if you're already on the verge of hypothyroidism—if your thyroid is subtly underperforming, or if you're on thyroid medication but the dosage is too low—then hypothyroid symptoms are likely to become prominent. These include fatigue, insomnia, acne, weight gain, and more (see Chapter 6). They also include symptoms you might already be accustomed to as a result of recycled hormones affecting your brain chemistry, such as depression, anxiety, and mood swings. However, the lack of adequate T3 can make what might otherwise be mild problems into major ones.

These ills can be difficult to recognize as thyroid-related because they're common aspects of PMS. But if you're experiencing an abrupt increase in their severity, or notice symptoms that have never happened before, then don't hesitate to get your thyroid tested (see Chapter 7).

When you get your blood taken for thyroid testing, be sure to tell your doctor where you're at in your cycle. That's because if you're in week three (when your hormones are peaking), your TSH level will be artificially raised a bit, making it appear higher than it really is the rest of the month. An experienced doctor will know this and take it into account when evaluating your test results.

Managing PMS

If testing reveals you're hypothyroid, then the most effective way you can reduce your PMS symptoms is by starting on thyroid medication and a healing diet (see Chapters 8, 9, and 18).

In addition, there are some simple things you can do to help your body prevent "used" estrogen hormones escaping from your liver or colon to recirculate and spread unhealthy byproducts.

First, cut down on coffee because caffeine helps estrogen escape the liver. It's also helpful to reduce *methylxanthines,* which are caffeine-like substances contained in chocolate and cocoa products.

Next, during the third week of your cycle when estrogen is peaking, consider taking 500 milligrams a day of *calcium d-glucarate.* This is an over-the-counter version of glucuronic acid, which is the protein your body uses to bind estrogen and keep it from leaving your colon. Calcium d-glucarate has virtually no side effects, and increasing your body's supply of glucuronic acid when it needs it most will help ensure the used estrogen stays in your colon until your body is ready to evict it via the stool.

When you look for calcium d-glucarate, don't mistakenly buy calcium gluconate. While their names are very similar, they're entirely different chemically and have entirely different effects.

You should also get more fiber in your colon. Fiber creates helpful bacteria that degrade used hormones into harmless chemicals (and, as a nice side effect, lower long-term risks of breast and ovarian cancer). Ideal for this purpose is *ground flax seed,* which you can buy in any health food store. Sprinkling a couple of tablespoons a day on top of cereal, smoothies, or soup during the third week of your cycle should do the trick. However, it's best to spread out the two tablespoons over a few meals instead of consuming it all at once; otherwise you might feel gassy and bloated until your body gets used to the ground flax seed.

In addition, take calcium during your third week—specifically, 1,300–1,500 milligrams per day of *calcium citrate* or *calcium citrate malate.* These calcium supplements help to inhibit hormone byproducts from acting on your brain cells.

If you're experiencing significant aches, pains, and cramping, over-the-counter anti-inflammatories such as ibuprofen and naproxen sodium are fine for most people if they're used short-term and at the recommended doses.

More generally, living healthy makes a big difference (see Chapters 18 and 20). Choose a balanced and nutritious diet, exercise regularly, get enough sleep, and engage in relaxing activities like spending time with friends. The stronger your body and mind are, the less vulnerable you'll be to hormonal byproducts.

Further, maintain a steady level of blood sugar. For example, don't skip meals, and eat balanced portions at each meal. Otherwise your adrenal glands might produce extra cortisol (see Chapter 14), which can add to the hormonal havoc of PMS.

If all these relatively simple measures aren't enough, though, you can additionally turn to your doctor for help.

For example, most PMS problems are caused by high levels of estrogen, while progesterone serves to block estrogen. If you're between 35 and 45, there's a chance your ovaries are secreting less progesterone, which means your body is effectively dealing with more estrogen, heightening your PMS.

It's a bad idea to self-medicate progesterone because it's not always needed, and it has significant side effects. Instead, ask a doctor who's an expert on PMS to check your hormone levels when you're around day 21 of your cycle and, if appropriate, prescribe a relevant dosage of progesterone for you.

If a thyroid problem is underlying your PMS issues, there's a good chance taking thyroid medication and following at least some of the solutions just described will allow you to live relatively happily with your PMS.

Infertility

One of life's most precious gifts is our ability to have children., And so one of the most heartbreaking ailments is the seeming inability to become pregnant.

Fertility problems sometimes stem from genetics or from age. But they're also often brought about by thyroid disease, which is easily treatable.

Hypothyroidism can cause infertility in several ways. First, thyroid hormones—and particularly T3—regulate the rate of cell growth. If your body doesn't have enough T3, it can inhibit the formation of the cells that support the egg, or *ovum*. A telltale sign of this occurring is irregular cycles.

Low T3 can also inhibit the production of progesterone, a hormone that's critical for ovulation. If this happens, your periods might stop altogether.

Another reason for infertility is a hormone called *prolactin,* which your body normally produces after you give birth to make your breasts lactate. Prolactin inhibits a sperm's ability to enter an egg, making it unlikely (though not impossible) that you'll get pregnant while nursing your newborn baby.

When your thyroid is underactive, your pituitary gland will release more TSH to stimulate the production of thyroid hormones. By coincidence, the pituitary is also in charge of making prolactin, and sometimes when it's churning out an unusually large amount of TSH, it'll inappropriately churn out prolactin, too.

In fact, having a high level of prolactin is one of the first noticeable signs of early thyroid disease. There usually won't be enough prolactin to make you lactate, but it could cause your periods to abruptly stop. And even if the latter doesn't occur, the prolactin will vastly decrease your chances of getting pregnant. Once you treat your hypothyroidism, though, your pituitary gland will stop making excessive TSH—and will simultaneously quit secreting prolactin.

Miscarriage

As painful as infertility is, even more tragic is a miscarriage. Unfortunately, thyroid problems greatly increase this risk, especially during the first trimester.

That's because for the first nine weeks your baby can't make thyroid hormones, and must rely entirely on your T4 and T3. Your baby's development can be severely impaired if your thyroid underproduces its hormones during this time and you don't take medication to correct the imbalance.

Further, if your hypothyroidism is caused by an autoimmune response, the increase in roving antibodies seeking foreign invaders to attack poses an additional danger to your baby.

It's common to be mildly hypothyroid before becoming pregnant and not be aware of it. It's also common to be latently hypothyroid—that is, have no symptoms at all, but be on the verge of thyroid disease. In either case, the upheaval of hormones that comes with pregnancy can nudge a thyroid from being barely healthy to ailing.

Pregnancy also brings vast changes to your immune system (because your body suddenly must consider not only your health but the health of your baby). As these transformations occur, they can spawn antibodies that attack both your thyroid and the thyroid hormones circulating in your blood, putting you into a hypothyroid state.

To make matters worse, hypothyroidism is far from obvious during pregnancy, because many of its symptoms—such as weight gain, fatigue, mood swings, and insomnia—can be attributed to the pregnancy itself.

Therefore, it's important for your doctor to order thyroid blood tests (including antibody tests) for you as soon as you discover that you're pregnant, and at least every 2–3 months after that.

If your thyroid is healthy, no harm will be done in checking it. But if it's started underperforming, then thyroid medication will quickly get your T3 level back to where it needs to be; and the medication will also lower your TSH level, which is likely to reduce antibody activity. This helps ensure your pregnancy remains on course.

Alternatively, you could become hyperthyroid during pregnancy. This is much less common; it happens only about 1 percent of the time. The main dangers are an increased heart rate for both you and your baby; a quicker metabolism, which can impair your body's ability to deliver sufficient nourishment to the baby; and a surplus of thyroid hormones, which poses a risk for your still-developing child. Because neither radiation nor anti-thyroid medications are safe for your baby, the best option for this situation is generally surgery to reduce your thyroid's size. If the result is an underactive thyroid, you can then take medication to get your thyroid hormone levels back to normal.

Postpartum Problems

Virtually everyone knows that a woman's body goes through massive hormonal and immune system changes during pregnancy. What not so many people consider is that it goes through similar transformations after giving birth. The conditions the body operated under for nine months no longer apply, and so it must make major adjustments.

For example, there are very high levels of the hormone progesterone during pregnancy, which helps thyroid hormones enter cells efficiently and so lowers the amount of work the thyroid has to do. After birth, however, there's an enormous drop in progesterone levels. This puts an abrupt and heavy strain on the thyroid, which suddenly needs to produce substantially more hormones than it was accustomed to for the previous nine months. This shock can trigger either a temporary or permanent thyroid problem.

One result is an autoimmune disorder called Graves' disease (see Chapter 10). The good news is there are more options for managing hyperthyroidism after pregnancy than during it (see Chapter 12).

Another disease that can result from changes to the immune system after pregnancy is postpartum thyroiditis (see Chapter 15). Postpartum thyroiditis is also an autoimmune disease, so doing antibody testing is especially important to detect it. This illness tends to end automatically after several months, and in the meantime is quite treatable. The trick is diagnosing it before a great deal of unnecessary suffering takes place.

Most common of all is hypothyroidism. This can cause unrelenting postpartum depression, as well as other severe symptoms. As terrible as its effects can be, however, it's the most easily treatable of these thyroid conditions (see Chapters 8, 9, and 18).

During the first six months after you give birth, you'll be faced with numerous challenges: learning to be a good parent, dealing with lack of sleep, becoming a magician at juggling multiple tasks, and so on. It's normal to feel physically run down and emotionally exhausted from it all. But if you're suffering from thyroid disease on top of that, you'll feel much worse than any mother should have to. If you suspect your thyroid is malfunctioning, don't hesitate to see your doctor. A simple blood test and some inexpensive pills may spare you from awful symptoms during what should be the happiest time of your life.

Perimenopause and Menopause

I realized that I was not alone. That 25 percent of perimenopausal and menopausal women experience some kind of issue with their thyroid at some time, and most women don't know that that's what it is.

—Oprah Winfrey on her hypothyroidism

Unlike thyroid disease, diagnosing menopause couldn't be more straightforward. There are no lab tests involved, and only one relevant symptom: whether you've had any periods over the past 12 months.

If you have, but your periods have been increasingly intermittent over time, then you're in *perimenopause*. This is a long-term stage during which your sex hormones—first *androgen* (which influences your sex drive and energy level), then progesterone, and finally estrogen—are steadily declining.

Specifically, around ages 38–42 your androgen levels significantly lower. This typically dampens your libido, slows your metabolic rate, and causes a general feeling of fatigue. It can also diminish the growth of lean body mass, forcing you to exercise more to avoid gaining fat (even as it makes you feel less energetic about exercising).

Around ages 38–45, progesterone levels decrease, which usually makes your PMS symptoms more severe and alters the timing of your cycles (causing you to miss periods, or at the other extreme experience mid-cycle bleeding).

At about ages 45–47, estrogen levels go down. The lessening stimulus of the uterine lining to thicken itself and cause your cycle to occur eventually leads to your periods stopping. It's during this phase that you start experiencing night sweats and hot flashes.

Your last menstrual cycle typically occurs within a few months of your 50th birthday (though if it happens a few years earlier or later, that's perfectly normal, too). And a year after that, you're officially in menopause.

All these phases involve major changes to your body's hormone activity, and that opens the door to your thyroid becoming strained and defective. When you consider the odds of getting thyroid disease go up with age anyway, it's understandable that many women become hypothyroid at some point during perimenopause.

Unfortunately, the hypothyroidism is often missed by doctors because its key symptoms—weight gain, fatigue, depression—can be attributed to perimenopause-related changes. That means it's your job to keep a special eye out for thyroid symptoms during this time of your life. If you have any reason to suspect hypo-thyroidism, see your doctor and get tested.

And even if you don't notice any symptoms, it's a good idea to get tested as part of your annual checkup once you begin perimenopause. Having a baseline reading on your thyroid hormone levels will make it easier for you and your doctor to later notice subtle indications that your thyroid is starting to underperform.
If your T4 and T3 levels remain normal but your TSH begins creeping up, try following the advice in Chapters 18 and 20; it might help you avoid progressing into hypothyroidism.

More broadly, if you have hypothyroidism or hyperthyroidism, or if you're on the verge of either disorder, read the next chapter, "Reversing Thyroid Disease Through Diet." You may find following its dietary recommendations to be at least as helpful to you as thyroid medication.

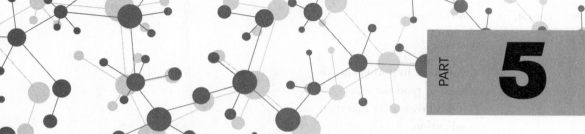

Healing Through Diet and Lifestyle

In this part, Chapter 18 provides you with dietary suggestions that could end up slowing, or even reversing, your thyroid disease.

In case you're having trouble losing weight, Chapter 19 gives you a program for shedding inches off your waist while also bolstering your liver.

And Chapter 20 helps you avoid toxins and stress, and embrace exercise.

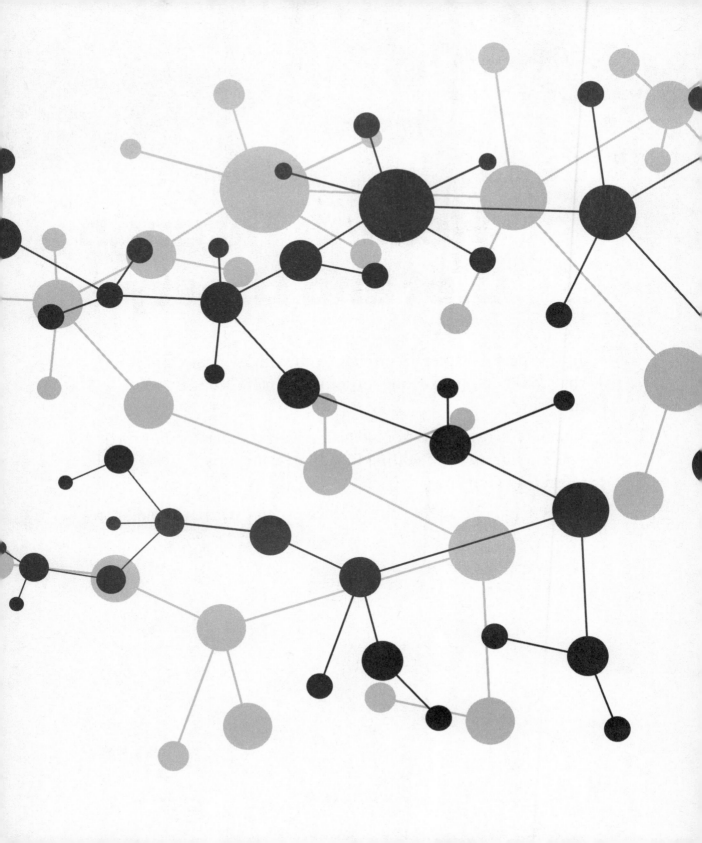

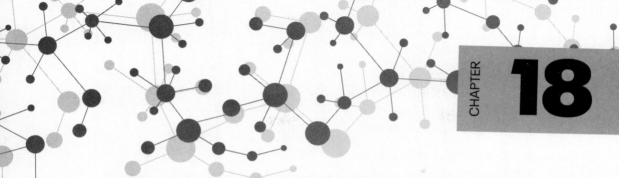

Reversing Thyroid Disease Through Diet

Medication isn't the only tool you can use to restore your health. At least as important is making health-driven choices about what you eat every day.

If you're in the early stage of a thyroid condition, changing your food habits in the ways this chapter suggests might stop the disease in its tracks.

But even if you've been suffering from thyroid disease for years, the diet that follows might slow the illness, and eventually even end it, allowing your thyroid the chance to finally heal.

Healing Through Iodine Management

There are many factors that might contribute to thyroid disease over which you have no control, such as your genetics, gender, age, and past exposure to radiation or viruses. But one major factor entirely within your control is your consumption of iodine.

In 2007, in recognition of the 100th year anniversary of Hakaru Hashimoto graduating from medical school, a number of researchers wrote papers pulling together all we've learned about thyroid disease in the past century. Their main conclusion was that excess iodine is behind more causes of thyroid disease than any other controllable factor.

How could a mineral that's essential to the thyroid's functioning also be the primary manageable trigger of thyroid disease?

For an analogy, imagine an automobile assembly line that can make up to 50 cars per day. Each morning a truck unloads the day's supply of tires. Because a car has four tires, the most the line can process are 200 tires daily.

If the truck fails to show up or brings too few tires, the factory can't meet its quota.

But what happens if the truck delivers more than 200 tires? There's no place to store them, and everyone stumbles over them. The workers start placing tires on top of the cars. If the assembly line stops, the tires build up even faster.

Something similar happens with iodine overloads.

From biochemical models, we know that above a low threshold, iodine intake turns on a mechanism that impairs thyroid activity and induces free radical damage.

From population studies, we know that regions with an iodine intake above 200 mcg per day have higher rates of thyroid disease. Plus people develop more thyroid disease after their countries fortify foods with iodine. This has happened in the United States, and more recently in Denmark.

Most startling, clinical trials have shown that regulating iodine intake can reverse thyroid disease for 78 percent of participants within three months!

In other words, based on available data, you might be able to restore your thyroid's health by temporarily switching to a low-iodine diet.

The studies concluding the latter sprang from an unexpected side effect of thyroid medical procedures. Patients are prescribed a low-iodine diet before having an iodine uptake scan or radioactive iodine ablation treatment, because depriving the thyroid of iodine for a while helps ensure it will quickly and fully suck in the new iodine of the procedure.

Researchers noticed a surprisingly high number of patients on low-iodine diets had spontaneous improvements in their thyroid function. This observation inspired multiple clinical trials to discover how often this happened.

Low-iodine diets that eliminated dairy, eggs, baked goods, and other high-iodine foods were studied for Hashimoto's disease, other hypothyroidism, subclinical (mild early stage) hypothyroidism, and Graves' disease.

In cases of Graves' disease, the results have been inconsistent. There are numerous case reports of beneficial responses, but studies have shown mixed results.

For every other condition, though, the results have been dramatic. Researchers found 60–80 percent of participants were able to reverse their Hashimoto's, other hypothyroidism, or subclinical hypothyroidism.

The period needed for reversal of disease was typically three months.

Participants in these studies were given no treatment other than diet; none had yet been placed on thyroid medication.

In many cases, those whose thyroid function didn't completely return to normal still saw big improvements. Had they continued the low-iodine diet, they might have regained their full health.

What can we infer from these studies?

We can say with confidence that for most thyroid disease patients, diet is as important, or more important, than thyroid medication.

And we can also say with confidence that eliminating dairy, eggs, baked goods, and other foods that these studies cut out is likely to be highly beneficial for most thyroid disease patients.

We can't be entirely certain of the reason. It's possible the types of foods these studies eliminated do harm to patients in ways we don't currently understand.

But the bottom line is that a low-iodine diet *works*. It's proved to be effective for most patients in mitigating or ending their thyroid disease. And because it consists of natural, healthy foods—fruits, vegetables, beans, legumes, nuts, seeds, gluten-free grains—it has no side effects.

Further, you don't have to choose between this diet and medication. In our experience, patients do fine being on the diet and thyroid meds at the same time.

We therefore recommend that you give the dietary changes detailed in this chapter a try. Aside from the inconvenience of changing your eating habits, you have nothing to lose...except, if all goes well, your thyroid disease.

Iodine's Narrow Safety Window

It's important to understand iodine isn't inherently bad for you. In fact, it's a fundamental building block for your thyroid's hormone production, so your thyroid couldn't function without it. The only problem with iodine is that we're consuming too much of it.

Unfortunately, it's easy to overdose on iodine. That's because it has the narrowest safety window of any nutrient.

By way of comparison, consider vitamin C. Those who consume too little vitamin C get scurvy. Those who take way too much vitamin C can get loose stools, possibly kidney stones, and other issues.

You can prevent scurvy by consuming as little as 10 mg (milligrams) of vitamin C daily; and the amount of Vitamin C that becomes harmful for most people is over 5,000 mg daily.

Between 10 mg and 5,000 mg is a very broad range of safety. In terms of physical mass, it's roughly the difference between a half-grain of rice and a full tablespoon of rice.

With iodine, the situation is completely different. For most adults, the safe range for iodine is 50–199 mcg (micrograms, or .001 mg) per day. (The main exception is if you're pregnant or breastfeeding; in this case, you should aim for around 220 mcg [when pregnant] or 290 mcg [when lactating] per day.)

To picture 50–199 mcg in physical terms, think of poppyseeds. If you had a pound of poppy seeds and took the time to count them out, you'd find it consisted of about 900,000 individual seeds.

Each poppyseed weighs around 300 mcg (micrograms). So in terms of mass, your safety margin for iodine would be roughly 17 percent to 66 percent of a single poppyseed.

That's a breathtakingly tiny safety margin.

We suspect the thyroid developed this way because iodine used to be scarce in most places, so it was important to be able to function on tiny amounts. In fact, there are still many areas in the world where people suffer from insufficient iodine.

But in dozens of developed countries, including the United States, the primary issue with iodine is that there's too much of it in foods, medications, and supplements.

Consider Going Vegan and Gluten-Free

What can you do to avoid overdosing on iodine?

First, start becoming aware of your iodine intake.

The standard American diet contains 200–1,000 mcg of iodine per day.

However, vegan diets are usually below 100 mcg. Vegan diets that are also gluten-free are often even lower (assuming they also avoid commercially baked gluten-free foods).

You can get all the protein you need on a vegan diet from dark green vegetables such as broccoli, organic kale, and organic spinach; and from lentils, beans, and grains such as quinoa. In fact, there's evidence plant protein is better for you than animal protein.

The only thing you're likely to run short of is vitamin B12, which you should take daily via a supplement.

So if you can manage to switch to a vegan and gluten-free diet for several months, it might have a dramatic positive impact on slowing or reversing your thyroid disease. That's especially true if you strive to primarily eat fresh (and ideally organic) vegetables and fruits—which carries a host of benefits even beyond thyroid health.

If you don't feel quite ready to go vegan, though, you can follow the guidelines directly below instead. They probably represent a big change from your usual eating habits too, but they don't forbid you from eating animal-based foods such as low-fat grass-fed beef, wild turkey, quail, and other low-fat meats.

A Low-Iodine Diet to Reverse Your Thyroid Disease

Each of us is unique, so there's no healing method that will work with equal effectiveness for everyone. But the chances are that if you heed the dietary guidelines below, you'll feel enormously better. And if you also stick to the recommendations in the rest of this chapter, you might slow or even reverse your thyroid disease.

The following are the main steps for changing your diet. These should be followed for at least three months, and be continued if you're experiencing positive results until your health is fully recovered:

. Stop taking any supplements that list iodine as an ingredient.

For example, it's a good idea to take multivitamins, but stick to ones that are iodine-free.

If you'd like a multivitamin specifically created for thyroid and adrenal disease patients, I formulated one in 2010 and update it twice a year based on the latest studies. You can find The Daily Reset Pack at DrChristianson.com/dailyresetpack.

Please note this rule about supplements does *not* apply to prescription thyroid medication. While T4 and T4/T3 meds such as Synthroid and Nature-Throid contain some iodine, if your doctor determines you need them, they're likely to do you much more good than harm.

Step 2. Cut out all dairy and all products that include dairy.

Dairy products are among the highest sources of iodine in a typical diet. That's in part because iodine is often fortified in the feed given to farm animals and is often used as a teat sanitizer in the milking process.

Therefore, remove all dairy from your diet. This includes:

O Milk (cow's milk, goat's milk, sheep's milk, etc.)

O Cheese

O Yogurt

O Ice cream

O Butter

O Anything else with dairy as an ingredient (carefully check all food labels)

For most people, this is a big ask. Cutting out dairy and the thousands of products that include it as an ingredient is an enormous lifestyle change.

But an even greater lifestyle change would be to end your thyroid disease.

Also, you can make up for any loss in nutrients by eating non-dairy foods rich in calcium. These include broccoli, organic kale, organic spinach, mustard and collard greens, okra, sweet potatoes, butternut squash, oranges, figs, chia seeds, sesame seeds, almonds, winged and white beans, lentils, amaranth, and a host of other natural, unprocessed foods that are great for you.

Another way to replace animal-based milk is to drink plant-based substitutes such as rice, almond, and coconut milk, which generally don't contain significant amounts of iodine. Many of these products used to be made with carrageenan and other seaweed extracts that were high in iodine. Nowadays, carrageenan has largely faded from use in non-dairy products. However, check ingredient labels to make sure carrageenan isn't included in anything you buy.

Step 3. Cut out all chicken, all eggs, and all products that include chicken or eggs.

Chickens are fed fish meal as a low-cost protein source. Fish meal is high in iodine, so the chickens end up with iodine, and so do the eggs they lay.

Therefore, remove all chicken and all eggs from your diet. This includes egg noodles, mayonnaise, hollandaise sauce; most cakes, pies, crepes, quiche, and waffles; and anything else with chicken or eggs as an ingredient.

As with dairy, carefully check all food labels to make sure you don't accidentally buy something with chicken or eggs in it.

Step 4. Avoid all commercial baked goods.

After dairy products and eggs, baked goods are the highest source of iodine in a typical diet. Iodine isn't present in grain or flour products, but various forms of iodine are often used in the commercial baking process.

Sometimes iodized dough conditioners might be listed on the label of baked goods. However, studies have shown products that don't list iodized dough conditioners can be high in iodine regardless, so the safe choice is to avoid all such products.

Therefore, remove all commercially baked goods from your diet. These include:

- Bread
- Bagels
- Rolls
- Cookies
- Croissants
- Danishes
- Pastries
- Pies

After you stop eating baked goods, you might find yourself feeling better beyond the lower iodine because many people don't do well with gluten.

As a substitute for commercial baked goods, it's fine to eat unprocessed grains. And it's also fine to use flour for your own home baking. However, pay attention to whether you feel worse after consuming gluten-based grains such as wheat, barley, and rye. If that occurs, simply stick to gluten-free grains, such as brown rice, quinoa, amaranth, sorghum, buckwheat, and teff.

Step 5. Avoid sea vegetables. They all contain extremely high amounts of iodine. In cultures that frequently eat sea vegetables, thyroid disease tends to run rampant.

All types of sea vegetables contain unsafe amounts of iodine. These include:

- Dulse
- Kelp
- Wakame
- Nori
- Hijiki
- Arame

Step 6. Avoid iodized salt. Most table salt is fortified with one-part potassium iodide per every 10,000 parts of salt. And even if they're not fortified, sea salt and pink Himalayan salt naturally contain notable amounts of iodine. Therefore, skip these salts.

Instead, you can use the following salts that are all free of significant amounts of iodine:

- Kosher salt, such as Diamond Crystal or Morton
- Non-iodized table salt
- Pickling salt
- Canning salt

Step 7. Avoid seafood with a high or unknown iodine content.

Seawater contains a significant level of iodine, so all life in the water has adapted to metabolizing iodine. This means fish, shellfish, mollusks, and other seafood all contain at least some iodine.

Seafood iodine content can vary by region, species, and season. But as a general guideline, saltwater fish and shellfish contain the highest amounts of iodine (roughly 330 mcg of iodine per 3.5 ounces of fish), while freshwater fish contain the least (roughly 66 mcg of iodine per 3.5 ounces of fish).

One other issue with seafood is it can contain mercury, which is far worse for your thyroid than too much iodine. So you must also take care to select only seafood known to be very low in mercury (see Chapter 20).

In other words, if you opt to eat seafood, choose carefully, and eat a limited amount.

Alternatively, if you cut seafood from your diet, be sure to consume omega 3 fats from other sources, such as flax seeds, chia seeds, and walnuts.

If you perform all seven of the steps above, it's likely to make a huge positive difference to your health.

To stack the odds even more in your favor, though, you should also follow the recommendations in the rest of this chapter, which include eating natural, unprocessed foods; eating foods appropriate for your metabolism; and consuming substances that are good for your thyroid.

Choosing Natural Versus Processed Foods

As explained in Chapter 5, your thyroid is especially sensitive to artificial chemicals and toxins. The more of them you consume, the more they're likely to accumulate in your thyroid and make it malfunction. Therefore, it's always a good idea to favor natural and organic foods over industrial and processed foods.

First, the processing of the food might involve harmful chemicals. For example, it was recently discovered that some manufacturers of corn syrup use mercury-based components, resulting in small amounts of mercury turning up in thousands of snacks, beverages, and other foods that include corn syrup in their ingredients.

Mercury is poisonous to the entire body, but it's especially harmful to the thyroid because it's chemically like iodine. That means your thyroid will absorb any mercury in your bloodstream and store it. Even though the amount in any single serving of food is minute, over time the mercury can accumulate to a level where it attracts the attention of your immune system and triggers a thyroid autoimmune disease such as Hashimoto's or Graves'.

If that scenario seems far-fetched, consider that corn growing is heavily government subsidized in the United States, making corn syrup exceptionally inexpensive...and included in just about every type of processed food imaginable. If you're straying from natural foods, your daily intake of corn syrup—and bits of mercury—may be a lot higher than you realize.

And beyond the toxins that are accidentally included in processed foods, you should be wary of the chemicals that are included intentionally.

Our air, water, offices, and homes are filled with artificial chemicals—there are more than 80,000 registered for commercial use in the United States alone.

Many of these substances haven't been around long enough for us to know what their long-term effects will be. Just as importantly, no one knows how you'll be affected by the combination of hundreds of chemicals in your daily life that have never been tested together.

So when you check the ingredients label of a processed food and see chemicals listed that no one's grandmother ever heard of, let alone would make a welcome part of a homemade meal, be aware that consuming that food is gambling with the health of both your thyroid and your whole body.

Along the same lines, you should avoid food grown through the process called *genetically modified organism*, or *GMO*. To save money, corporations have altered the genes of what used to be food staples—corn, soy, sugar beets, peas, canola—to make them easier to grow and resistant to pests. No one knows for sure what effects unnatural genetic designs for repelling bugs has on the human beings eating them. But considering the skyrocketing levels of disease in the United States, the safe course is to steer clear of GMO. That means avoiding all products with corn, soy, beet sugar, peas, or canola oil unless they're labeled as non-GMO or GMO-free.

In addition, avoid additives that there's reason to believe are terrible for you, such as MSG (often hidden in ingredients lists as "natural flavors") and artificial sweeteners.

One grim upside to this situation is that it's made a bit easier identifying what you should avoid. When you read a food product's label and spot canola oil, corn syrup, or "natural flavors" as an ingredient, that's all you need to know to return that product to the shelf.

In addition, when possible, buy organic food. Pesticides that kill insects aren't going to be kind to your body either.

Alternatively, if you can't manage to always buy organic, commit to at least doing so for strawberries, spinach, and kale, which are typically loaded with more pesticides than any other produce.

Also, when you can't buy organic, thoroughly wash your produce before eating it. That's likely to remove about 80 percent of its pesticides.

Choosing Foods Fitting Your Metabolism

Another way to eat smart is to be aware of which foods are a good fit for your metabolic rate (see Chapter 1). If you're hypothyroid, your insulin will be less effective at lowering blood sugar and helping convert it into energy. You'll therefore want to eat foods that can put your body into "calorie-burning mode" rather than "food-storage mode."

For example, high-fiber fruits and vegetables (pears, apples, bananas, carrots, Brussels sprouts), legumes (pinto beans, chickpeas, lentils), and high-protein foods (broccoli, organic kale and spinach) will stay in your stomach for a while before moving on to your small intestines, and then your bloodstream. This allows for gradual digestion and low releases of blood sugar, requiring relatively little insulin; and it puts your body into a "calorie-burning mode" that's likely to turn the food directly into energy.

Conversely, sugary low-fiber foods (cookies, donuts) and starchy foods (pasta, white rice) speed through your system, spending only a little time in your stomach before being converted to blood glucose. Your body reacts to this sugar jolt by releasing a lot of insulin, putting you into a "storage mode" likely to turn a fair amount of the food into fat.

You can learn how your body will react to a food by checking its *glycemic load,* which is a measure of how quickly your blood glucose level will rise after eating it. If you're trying to lose weight, then you'll favor foods with a glycemic load under 10, and ideally under 6.

If you're hypothyroid, also try to avoid foods high in saturated fats (fatty beef, pork, lamb, dark meat poultry). First, they're calorie intensive. And second, they make your cell membranes resistant to insulin. That means you'll need more insulin than usual to process the same amount of glucose; and because your insulin is already inefficient right now, such foods make a bad situation worse and are likely to turn directly into body fat.

Helping Your Thyroid Work

There are two chemicals that have special importance to your thyroid. The first is iodine, which we've discussed at length in this chapter. The second is selenium, which plays a role in your body's conversion of T4 to T3 (see Chapter 1). If a blood test turns up a selenium shortage, you can easily solve it by eating one Brazil nut daily. (Don't eat more than one a day regularly, though, as too much selenium is bad for you.)

If you need to take thyroid medication for hypothyroidism, seriously consider desiccated thyroid. In addition to such benefits as being the only medication to provide all four thyroid hormones (see Chapter 3), natural thyroid might boost healing. That's because when you consume an animal's gland, the parts of it that aren't digested will be transported by your immune system to the corresponding gland in your body to strengthen and help rebuild it.

Just in case your thyroid issue is at least partially being caused by an infection, consider trying over-the-counter antiviral/antibacterial supplements to see if they make you feel better. Popular supplements include vitamin C (1,000–2,000 mg, taken with food to avoid upsetting your stomach), cat's claw, L-lysine, lemon balm, and goldenseal (taken at the dosages recommended on their respective labels).

What *Can* I Eat?

Whether you switch to a vegan diet or follow the alternative recommendations in this chapter, changing your life-long dietary habits is hard.

At first blush, you might feel as if we've left almost nothing for you to eat.

However, the truth is that you still have many wonderful options.

Specifically, you can still eat all fruits, all vegetables (except GMO versions), all nuts, all seeds, all beans, and all legumes.

You can also eat gluten-free grains such as brown rice, quinoa, amaranth, sorghum, buckwheat, and teff.

If you go the non-vegan route, you can eat low-fat grass-fed beef, wild turkey, quail, and other low-fat meats that are also low in iodine.

Plus you can still eat seafood, as long as you carefully choose only low-mercury and low-iodine varieties in small portions.

If you still feel that's not enough variety, please Google around for vegan recipes. You'll discover thousands of them. Many of them are for dishes you never dreamed of...and that you'll probably find delicious.

Also keep in mind this lifestyle change doesn't have to be permanent. It's a temporary diet designed to ease or end your thyroid disease. Depending on a variety of factors, you might need to be on it for three months, six months, or longer. If the diet proves effective for you, we're hoping you become increasingly motivated to stay on it as you continue getting better.

And speaking of timing: If you're already taking thyroid medication, we recommend you get your TSH, free T4, and free T3 blood levels tested after your first month on the diet. If your thyroid starts functioning better, you might need to change your medication to a lower dosage. In addition, this will put your doctor on notice to keep a close eye on your progress.

Stick with the diet for at least three months, and then get tested again. You and your doctor can then decide whether the diet is benefitting you; if so, how much progress you've made; and roughly how many more months you should stay on it to restore your health.

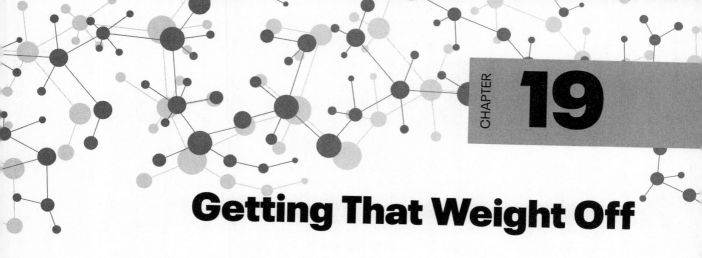

Getting That Weight Off

If you've been hypothyroid and then prescribed medication, you may have experienced a doctor telling you, "You can go ahead and take that extra weight off now. Good luck." Good luck indeed.

For a fortunate 20 percent of patients, the newly added pounds are magically shed once their metabolisms are restored. But if you're like most people, all your stable condition will do is give you the *opportunity* to lose weight. You'll need to actively work at getting your body back in shape. The best advice for doing so has always been "Eat less and exercise more," and we heartily echo that. But this chapter also offers some suggestions you might not have heard before to help you succeed.

Focusing on Fiber

As explained in Chapter 18, foods that digest slowly and gradually, rather than racing from your stomach to your bloodstream, create less of a sugar jolt and less need for insulin. This puts your body into a calorie-burning mode that converts the food into energy (versus a food-storage mode that turns it into fat).

One of the best ways to achieve this effect is to choose foods with lots of fiber. Fiber ensures what you eat stays around a while in your stomach and small intestines, making it more likely the food will be burned right away as fuel.

In addition, fiber gives you a feeling of being filled up and satisfied on smaller portions of food, which in turn, makes it easier for you to eat less. And fiber makes you want to drink more water, which also fills you up and enables you to get by with less food.

Beyond aiding weight loss, fiber helps your intestines eliminate waste efficiently. The health benefits from this include flushing out toxins that are bad for your thyroid, preventing constipation (which is a hypothyroid symptom), and guarding against digestive diseases, diabetes, and some cancers. If you adjust to it gradually—say, adding 3–4 grams to your diet every few days to avoid bloating—there's really no downside to fiber.

According to nutritional experts, for overall health women should eat at least 25 grams of fiber a day and men should eat at least 38 grams a day. For the purposes of weight loss, it's a good idea to strive for 40 grams a day (for both genders).

If you're typical, you currently eat less than 15 grams of fiber daily. But that's good news because it means your diet has lots of room for improvement.

Delicious high fiber foods include:

○ Legumes (lentils, navy beans, black beans, pinto beans, adzuki beans)

○ Whole grains (brown rice, quinoa, amaranth, sorghum, buckwheat)

○ Vegetables (broccoli, organic kale and spinach, eggplant, Brussels sprouts, carrots)

○ Fruits (apples, plums, pears, peaches, mangoes, kiwi)

○ Berries (blackberries, raspberries, blueberries)

○ Nuts (pecans, pistachios, hazelnuts, Brazil nuts)

○ Seeds (almonds, flax seeds, sunflower seeds, pumpkin seeds)

Certain high-fiber foods are especially helpful because they also aid in detoxifying you by flushing unhealthy chemicals and other wastes from your system. Examples include cilantro, brown rice, flax seeds, and organic spinach.

Another great fiber source is adzuki beans (also called aduki beans), which are small reddish beans that typically have a white tip or streak, and are popular in China and Japan. They're packed with magnesium, which plays many vital roles in the body, including aiding thyroid function. Plus if you're swinging between hypothyroidism and hyperthyroidism, magnesium is a terrific low-impact remedy for stabilizing your heart rate.

In a nutshell, if counting calories isn't working for you, you may be able to lose weight even more effectively by counting fiber grams.

How Is Your Metabolism?

A lot of people have a metabolism that doesn't work quite right. They find they can lose weight only if they starve themselves or perform extreme amounts of exercise. Such approaches aren't sustainable, nor are they safe.

A healthy metabolic rate depends on the liver functioning well. But researchers estimate as many as 100 million Americans have *fatty liver disease* (excess fat in the liver). This condition hampers the liver's ability to work efficiently. (Over time, it can also seriously endanger your health; see Chapter 21.)

Making things more complicated is that your liver needs nutrients to do its job. If you eat less, you may prevent your liver from getting the nutrients it needs to get rid of the fats stored within it.

People with thyroid disease are especially prone to the sort of liver issues that lead to weight loss resistance and render conventional diets ineffective. Years of working with thyroid disease patients taught me a new approach was necessary.

The Metabolism Reset Diet

The doctors at Integrative Health and I developed a diet to help those with resistance to weight loss. Our initial goal was actually to combat diabetes. However, we found that in addition to treating that disease, the diet helped patients who couldn't lose weight before to shed inches off their waists. We then tried it with thyroid patients who were unable to lose weight and found it was effective for them, too.

The program is based on a simple concept: consume adequate protein, but limit your fats and carbohydrates. At the same time, include nutrients, such as resistant starch, that help to regulate blood sugar. This approach allows you to hold onto muscle mass and also avoid an out-of-control appetite while you're getting rid of stored fat.

The program is designed to make most of your weight loss come from fat around and inside your organs. You might experience a dramatic shrinkage of inches around your waist within the first few weeks.

Each day's menu consists of the following:

○ A plant-based protein shake for breakfast

○ A plant-based protein shake for lunch

○ A relatively conventional but portion-controlled meal for dinner

○ Unlimited snacks of vegetables throughout the day

This way of eating is probably different from what you're used to. After about a week, though, you might find it becoming an easy habit. It lets you spend less time on food and gives you more energy.

The following sections detail each part of the diet.

Making Your Shakes Overview

Shakes consist of a plant-based protein, resistant starch, seeds, flavorings, and optionally a sweetener. The group of possible ingredients is relatively small, but you can combine them in scores of different ways. If you buy all the ingredients at the same time, you'll have the freedom of making whatever type of shake you're in the mood for each day.

Any kind of blender can be used to make your shakes. However, some ingredients will have the best texture when processed by a high-power blender such as Vitamix, NutriBullet, Ninja, or Blendtec.

Mix and drink your first shake within an hour of waking up. (If you're on thyroid medication, take your pill as soon as you wake up and then make your shake an hour later.) Once you blend the ingredients, the taste and texture of your shake will be good for several hours at room temperature (or a full day if insulated and refrigerated).

If you get hungry easily, drink your shake more slowly using a reusable wide straw. The process will take longer and give you more of a chance to fill up.

If you want your shakes as fresh as possible, and also enjoy variety, make one type of shake in the morning for breakfast and a different type of shake in the afternoon for lunch.

Alternatively, if you prefer to save some time and effort, or if you don't have access to your kitchen in the afternoon, use twice as many ingredients in the morning to make the same shake for both breakfast and lunch. Store the shake for lunch in an insulated non-plastic container (e.g., a glass bottle or thermos), and refrigerate it until you're ready to start drinking it.

When choosing the ingredients for each shake, make flavor a high priority. You won't drink it if you don't like it.

Shake Ingredients

A shake is made up of a plant-based protein, resistant starch, seeds, and flavorings. Details about each ingredient appear below.

Plant-Based Protein

Start your shake with a plant-based protein base that has no artificial ingredients, no common allergens, no refined sugar, no GMO, and at least 23 grams of protein per serving. Here are some suggestions:

○ Pea protein powder (make sure it's labeled non-GMO)

○ Pumpkin seed powder

○ Brown rice powder

○ Sacha inchi powder

○ Plant protein blends (e.g., non-GMO pea protein and rice protein)

These ingredients can be used for almost any protein shake recipe you find in a book or on the web. The recipe might specify a different type of protein base, but feel encouraged to substitute and see if you like the result.

Aquafaba

The enjoyment of shakes has as much to do with texture as it does with flavor. The water from beans—which is called *aquafaba*—has no taste, but it's an excellent thickener for texture; and it's also a great source of resistant starch.

The quickest way to get aquafaba is to use the liquid from a can of chickpeas or white beans (navy, northern, or cannellini). Make sure the cans are BPA free, with no ingredients other than the beans.

Drain the liquid from the can and use it in your shake. In addition, store the chickpeas or white beans in your refrigerator, because you can use them for the next two days in your shakes (see the next section).

For a fresher alternative, though, make the aquafaba yourself. Here's how:

1. Place 1 pound of dried chickpeas (approximately 2 cups) into a large fine-mesh colander. Pick through the beans, discarding any that aren't mature. Rinse well for 2 minutes.

2. Pour the chickpeas into a large jar and cover them with 5 cups of water. Close the lid, and let the jar sit for 12 hours or overnight.

3. Transfer the chickpeas and liquid into a saucepan. Make sure the chickpeas are covered by at least one inch of water. (Add water if necessary.)

4. Bring the chickpeas and water mixture to a boil. Reduce the heat until the chickpeas are at a low simmer. Cook until soft. This might take between 40 to 60 minutes, and you might need to add water.

5. The resulting liquid should be about the same thickness as the aquafaba from a can of chickpeas. If it seems too thin, place the liquid back on your stovetop and simmer until the desired consistency is reached.

If you don't happen to care for aquafaba, or you crave variety, you can use frozen bananas or unsweetened flax milk as substitutes. Use bananas or flax milk as substitutes only, though, not in addition to aquafaba.

Don't use cow's milk, almond milk, coconut milk, rice milk, or any other type of milk other than unsweetened flax milk.

Resistant Starch

To make your shake's resistant starch, use ½ cup of aquafaba along with any one of the following ingredients:

- ○ Green banana flour (¼ cup)
- ○ Frozen banana with peel (½)
- ○ Non-GMO pea starch (1 serving)

○ White beans (¼ cup)

○ Navy beans (¼ cup)

○ Northern beans (¼ cup)

○ Cannellini beans (¼ cup)

It might seem odd to include beans in a smoothie. But white beans are the highest in resistant starch, and have a neutral flavor. They'll give your shake a rich and creamy texture, and cause your body to absorb the shake's ingredients more slowly, which will keep you feeling full longer.

Seeds

Include ½ tablespoon of any of the following seeds in your shake:

○ Chia seeds

○ Flax seeds

○ Hemp seeds

○ Sesame seeds

○ Sunflower seeds

Flavorings

Include as much as you like of any of the following flavorings in your shake:

○ Cinnamon

○ Ginger

○ Luo han guo/monk fruit extract (a sweetener)

○ Natural extracts (vanilla, almond, chocolate)

○ Food-grade essential oils (lemon, wild orange, peppermint)

Play around with the ingredients to make shakes you think you'll enjoy. After you've experimented with 5–10 recipes, pick your favorites, and stick with those for the next week or so to get you through the initial adjustment period.

Once the diet feels less like a novelty and more like a comfortable habit, experiment with ingredients as much as you like to discover the shakes that are most satisfying for you. You can also Google vegan protein shake recipes to give you more ideas, as long as you don't stray from the list of ingredients above.

Midmorning Snacks

If you crave snacks, you can have as much as you want of the veggies and seasonings listed below. You can mix them in whatever combinations you like, in either raw or cooked form.

You'll probably find these snacks essential during your first few days on the program. After that, you might become indifferent to them. If that happens, it's perfectly fine, as the snacks are optional and should be eaten only when you feel like it.

Unlimited Veggies

O Alfalfa sprouts

O Arugula

O Artichoke

O Artichoke hearts

O Asparagus

O Baby bok choy

O Bamboo shoots

O Bean sprouts

O Bok choy

O Broccoli

O Brussels sprouts

- O Butter lettuce
- O Cabbage
- O Carrots
- O Cauliflower
- O Celery
- O Celery root
- O Chicory greens
- O Collard greens
- O Crookneck squash
- O Cucumber
- O Daikon
- O Eggplant
- O Endive
- O Escarole
- O Fennel
- O Garlic
- O Ginger
- O Green beans
- O Green leaf lettuce
- O Green onions
- O Green peppers
- O Jicama
- O Kale (organic)
- O Kohlrabi
- O Leeks

- O Lemon juice
- O Lime juice
- O Mushrooms
- O Okra
- O Onions
- O Pea pods
- O Pumpkin
- O Radicchio
- O Radishes
- O Red leaf lettuce
- O Red peppers
- O Romaine lettuce
- O Rutabaga
- O Scallions
- O Snow peas
- O Spaghetti squash
- O Spinach (organic)
- O Summer squash
- O Swiss chard
- O Tomato
- O Tomatillos
- O Turnip greens
- O Water chestnuts
- O Watercress
- O Zucchini

Unlimited Seasonings

- Non-iodized sea salt
- White vinegar
- Apple cider vinegar
- Red wine vinegar
- Black pepper
- Mustard
- Tamari soy sauce (organic and MSG-free)
- Coconut aminos
- Ginger
- Garlic
- Turmeric
- Cumin
- Basil
- Oregano
- Thyme

Some of these are easy grab-and-go foods, such as baby carrots. But if you're creative about it, you can craft delicious and filling dishes such as homemade tomato sauce with mushrooms served over spaghetti squash and zucchini noodles.

Lunch

If you make your breakfast and lunch shake at the same time, store the shake for lunch in an insulated non-plastic container (e.g., a glass bottle or thermos) and refrigerate it until you're ready to start drinking it. Otherwise, make your lunch shake fresh in the afternoon.

Start drinking your lunch shake within 4–6 hours of your breakfast shake. The goal is to have a solid dose of protein three times daily to supply your liver with the amino acids it needs to detoxify, and to keep your body from breaking down your muscles.

Instead of gulping down your lunch shake, make lunch an event. Go to a new location, ideally outdoors. Put your phone away and focus on your meal, allowing yourself at least 15–20 minutes to complete it.

Much of hunger is psychological. When you don't make a meal your top mental focus, it won't satisfy you as much. It takes some time and focus for your brain to register the fact that you've just had a meal.

If you occasionally have to attend a business or social gathering for lunch, or you simply crave a change of pace, flip lunch and dinner. In other words, order food for lunch, then have your shake in the evening in place of your usual dinner. You can do this up to two times a week as a harmless variation.

Midafternoon Snacks

Your midafternoon snack options are identical to your midmorning snacks. If you'll be on the go in the afternoon, plan ahead by preparing and bringing the snacks with you.

Again, the snacks aren't mandatory, and they might become much less important to you after your first week. But if you want them, eat as much of them as you like.

Dinner

For dinner, not only do you get to eat a solid meal, you get to eat well. This meal is likely to make you feel fuller and sleep better. It also makes it easier for you to stick with the program and enjoy its benefits.

Your dinner consists of a protein, resistant starch, high-nutrient veggies, fats that are good for you, and seasonings. Once you grow familiar with the ingredients, you'll be able to make an unlimited number of tasty dishes with them.

Protein

The centerpiece of your dinner is your protein. Try to use a different protein food from one day to the next, both so that you never get bored and to ensure your body is taking in a broad range of nutrients.

Include a 4–6 ounce serving of any one of the following foods:

- O Broccoli (unlimited)
- O Wild turkey
- O Freshwater fish
- O Lean grass-fed beef
- O Quail
- O Tempeh (non-GMO)
- O Tofu (non-GMO)

For the sake of variety, you can add edamame (non-GMO only) or spirulina to your protein.

Resistant Starch

The resistant starch in your dinner will help fill you up and make you feel satisfied. It'll also supply you with a full spectrum of fiber.

Include one serving of any one of the following foods:

- O Boiled potatoes (1 cup)
- O Sweet potato/yam (1 cup)
- O Plantain (1 cup)
- O Peas (1 cup)
- O Legumes (cooked, ¾ cup)
- O Lentils
- O Garbanzos

O Navy beans

O Northern beans

O Black beans

O Lotus seed

O White beans

O Split peas

O Brown rice

O Buckwheat

O Quinoa

O Amaranth

O Sorghum

O Teff

Nutrient-Rich Veggies

High-nutrient, low-fuel veggies will make up most of your dinner's volume. All the veggies below are good for you, but make a point of including at least one of the following veggies that are especially helpful for your liver: broccoli, cauliflower, cabbage, carrots, garlic, onions, parsnips, parsley.

Include as much as you like of the following veggies:

O Artichokes

O Arugula

O Asparagus

O Beans, Green

O Beans, Yellow

O Beans, Wax

O Beet greens

O Beets

O Bell peppers

O Bok choy

O Broccoli

O Broccoli rabe

O Broccolini

O Brussels sprouts

O Cabbage

O Carrots

O Cauliflower

O Celery

O Collards greens

O Cucumber

O Dandelion greens

O Eggplant

O Endive

O Escarole

O Fennel

O Garlic

O Ginger

O Green onions

O Jicama

O Kale (organic)

O Leeks

O Mixed greens

- O Mushrooms
- O Mustard greens
- O Okra
- O Onions
- O Peppers
- O Pumpkin
- O Radicchio
- O Radishes
- O Red peppers
- O Rhubarb
- O Romaine
- O Shallot
- O Snow peas
- O Spaghetti squash
- O Spinach (organic)
- O Sprouts (all varieties)
- O Summer squash
- O Swiss chard
- O Tomatoes
- O Turnip greens
- O Watercress

Good Fats

Your dinner should also include, in limited amounts, fats that are good for you. You'll get these fats in the form of nuts and seeds, or as cooking oil. Add the latter at the final stages of your cooking because oil often is heat stable.

Use 1–2 teaspoons of any of the following oils in your cooking:

O Extra Virgin Olive oil (EVOO)

O Sesame oil

O Walnut oil

Alternatively, include 1–2 tablespoons of any the following nuts and seeds:

O Almonds

O Flax seeds

O Macadamia nuts

O Pecans

O Pistachios

O Sunflower seeds

O Walnuts

Herbs and Seasonings

The right mix of herbs and seasonings will help make your meal delicious. The ones listed below are also good for you, and you can include as much of them as you like:

O Asafetida

O Basil

O Black pepper

O Cardamom

O Chives

O Coriander

O Cumin

O Fennel

O Galangal

- Garlic
- Ginger
- Lemongrass
- Mint
- Nutmeg
- Oregano
- Paprika
- Rosemary
- Tarragon
- Thyme
- Turmeric

Condiments

You can also spice up the flavor of your dinner with condiments. However, beware of a manufacturer sneaking in things that are bad for you, such as MSG (hidden under such labeling as "natural flavors") and items that are GMO. Instead, look for labels that show the condiment to be organic and non-GMO.

That noted, you can use the following condiments in moderation:

- Ketchup (organic and sugar-free)
- Mustard (organic)
- Tamari (organic and non-GMO; use sparingly because of high sodium)
- Toasted sesame oil
- Ume plum vinegar
- Apple cider vinegar

Once you grow familiar with the program, you can optionally swap in foods you love that aren't on the lists above, as long as they fit with the program's goals. However, try only one such change at a time, and pay close attention to see if the new addition ends up making you feel worse or leads to a sudden increase in weight.

If you'd like to learn more about the program, visit MetabolismResetDiet.com or ThyroidResetDiet.com. You can also find related resources at ThyroidResetDiet. com/resources.

The T2 Factor

If you're on thyroid medication but the weight still isn't coming off (despite your best efforts), the problem could be a lack of T2. As explained in Chapter 3, most doctors treat hypothyroidism by automatically prescribing Synthroid or its generic version levothyroxine. These are fine medications, but they include only T4. Desiccated thyroid medications, such as Nature-Throid and Armour Thyroid, are the only available sources for T2 aside from the thyroid itself.

Until recently, it was assumed T2 did nothing important, so drug manufacturers weren't motivated to create chemical versions of it. Then it occurred to researchers that if the thyroid makes T2, there's probably a good reason for it. Their subsequent studies have indicated T2 plays a significant role in weight loss.

Specifically, preliminary results show T2 speeds the rate at which your body's cells retrieve and break down fats, which are the first steps in burning your body fat and converting it into energy. T2 also helps offset insulin's effect of putting the body into food-storage mode rather than calorie-burning mode. And T2 facilitates the conversion of T4 into T3, which raises overall metabolism.

Further, studies indicate that T4 seldom converts down to T2.

So if you're on thyroid medication that's exclusively T4, and you care about losing weight, you should seriously consider switching to desiccated thyroid.

This chapter has described a program that might help you shed fat dramatically. Just as important to your health, though, is avoiding hazards to your thyroid, cutting down on stress, and exercising. These subjects are covered next.

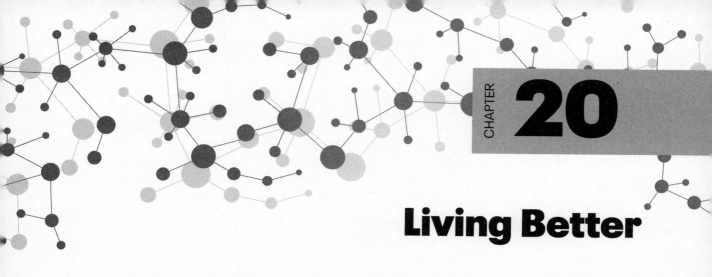

20

Living Better

Chapter 18 discussed toxins and excesses in foods that have the potential to disrupt your thyroid. Unfortunately, there are other sources of dangerous chemicals you also need to be aware of. In this chapter, we describe some of the most notable environmental threats to your thyroid and ways you can avoid them.

In addition, we discuss how to mitigate the intangible toxin *stress*, which can wear down your thyroid as well as the rest of your body.

Finally, we point out some of the immense benefits of exercise.

We hope the suggestions that follow help you enjoy a longer, healthier, and happier life.

Thyroid Threats

As explained in Chapter 1, your thyroid is designed to suck every bit of iodine out of your bloodstream and store it until needed. The problem is your thyroid will also draw in artificial chemicals that make their way into your bloodstream and that your body was never designed to handle.

While this can happen with a number of chemicals, there are certain ones to which your thyroid is especially vulnerable because their composition is very similar to that of iodine. Your thyroid will absorb every molecule of these it can find and permanently store them. As they accumulate, they can interfere with your thyroid's functioning by displacing iodine; doing direct physical damage to your thyroid; and/or attracting the attention of your immune system, leading to an autoimmune disease such as Hashimoto's or Graves'.

The three substances most likely to threaten your thyroid because of their chemical resemblance to iodine are mercury, perchlorate, and fluoride.

Mercury

Mercury is a dangerous poison found in minute amounts in thousands of processed foods. Mercury is also present in fish. Chapter 18 explained why you should pay attention to a seafood's level of iodine. It's additionally wise to refrain from consuming fish likely to have the highest levels of mercury—which are swordfish, thresher sharks, and marlin.

Also worrisome is tuna. While its mercury levels aren't as high as those of the somewhat exotic fish just mentioned, tuna is eaten so frequently that its mercury can accumulate at an alarming rate. And counterintuitively, it's the highest-quality tuna that poses the greatest risk. That's because top-grade tuna comes from larger, older fish, and they're the ones that have lived long enough to build up the most mercury in their bodies. You're at lowest risk eating flaked "light" tuna; at moderate risk with albacore; at significant risk with the "tuna steak" grade...and you probably shouldn't even think about consuming sushi-grade tuna beyond rare occasions.

If you suspect you're suffering from mercury poisoning, talk to your doctor about getting tested for it. The process involves taking a dose of mercury chelating medicine—which removes heavy metals from your body—and then providing your urine. By measuring the amount of mercury that comes out of your body, a lab can estimate how much mercury is stored in your thyroid.

Perchlorate

Perchlorate is another chemical similar enough to iodine to fool your thyroid. While not as poisonous as mercury, perchlorate is a byproduct of rocket fuel production, so it's hardly people friendly. Studies have found even low levels of perchlorate can interfere with the thyroid's ability to make hormones, leading to hypothyroidism.

Perchlorate has been found in the water supplies of more than 35 American states. If you believe it's an issue in your area, you can buy high-quality bottled water or you can install a special filter that purifies your tap water. Most conventional filters won't do the job in this case, but a reverse osmosis system designed to trap perchlorate will. This can cost as little as $150, plus $20–$30 for filter changes once or twice a year.

Fluoride

Like mercury and perchlorate, fluoride is chemically like iodine. The more fluoride your thyroid absorbs, the less room there is for iodine, and the more likely it is that the fluoride will block iodine from your thyroid's hormone construction sites.

The amounts of fluoride you're exposed to in toothpaste, or from your city or town adding it to your local water supply, are too small to have a significant impact on your thyroid.

However, it's a genuine problem if you're in an area that has toxic amounts of fluoride in the soil and that fluoride turns up in your water supply. Fluoride at high levels is so effective at reducing T4 and T3 production that it's used as a treatment for hyperthyroidism (see Chapter 12). If you're on the verge of being hypothyroid, a high level of fluoride can push you over the edge. And if you're already hypothyroid, it can make your condition even worse. So if you suspect there's excessive fluoride in your tap water, buy a system to filter it out.

Cutting Down on Chemicals

While mercury, perchlorate, and fluoride are the best-known threats to your thyroid, they're far from the only ones. Any modern artificial chemical, or combination of chemicals, could have an unexpectedly adverse effect. Your best defense is to avoid as many of them as possible.

For example, a 2010 study found people with high levels of the chemical *perfluorooctanoic acid,* or *PFOA,* are twice as likely to have thyroid disease. PFOA is used in nonstick Teflon cookware, microwave popcorn bags, stain-resistant carpet and fabric coatings, and certain cleansers.

Most of these are products you can live without. For example, you can use enamel-coated cast iron pans instead of Teflon, and you can microwave air-pop popcorn using brown paper lunch bags.

As for cleansers, you should ideally buy organic versions that contain no harmful chemicals. These include Dr. Bronner's Sal Suds, KD Gold, and a line of green products from Seventh Generation.

You can also use old-fashioned, but still effective, solutions such as white vinegar and water for cleaning windows; weakly brewed black tea for mirrors; lemon juice or vinegar for most stains; club soda for carpet stains; and cornmeal for spills.

Similarly, you should choose organic products in place of:

O Artificial pesticides, especially when spraying inside your house (try boric acid, which is nontoxic).

O Chemical-based cosmetics and body care products.

O Insecticide- and herbicide-saturated wines and beers.

Most chemical engineers are never trained in toxicology, which means they invent new chemicals without deep knowledge of the potential effects on people. This has caused untold misery. In response, a green, organic movement has developed that allows you to live a safer, more natural, and healthier life. Don't hesitate to join it.

Shrinking Stress

Stress can have just as negative an impact on you as chemical toxins. A common result of our fast-paced lives, stress triggers an adrenaline rush that raises your heart rate, quickens your breath, and moves your blood away from your organs toward your skeletal muscles, readying you to respond by either fighting or fleeing.

This worked great when our ancestors regularly faced off against tigers and rival tribes. However, it's not as helpful when you're being criticized by your boss or stuck in a traffic jam.

Stress impairs your digestive system, your immune system, and your body's ability to repair itself. If sustained for a long time, it'll wear you down and make you sick.

You don't have to helplessly suffer, though. There are a number of things you can try to reduce stress:

O **Avoid the person stressing you out.** If it's a friend or colleague, be polite but firm. If it's your manager and the stress is unending, consider finding another job.

○ **Avoid the situation stressing you out.** For example, if standing in line is aggravating, get your chores done during non-peak hours or hire someone to do them for you.

○ **Say "no."** If you really don't want to do something, then don't.

○ **Talk it out.** If it's not possible to say "no," then tactfully express your frustration. Maybe a compromise can be reached.

○ **Focus on what fulfills you.** If you love spending time with your family, figure out ways to do more of that. If you dream of being an actor, take classes and join a community theater. If you have a book burning inside you, carve out an hour each day to work on it (or hire Hy to help you via BookProposal.net). As Joseph Campbell put it, "follow your bliss."

○ **Adjust your perspective.** Sometimes if you decide to not let something bother you, it won't.

○ **Do something calming.** Meditation, yoga, visualization, gardening, or listening to music...whatever relaxes you is good.

○ **Breathe.** Breathe in through your nose for seven seconds, and then breathe out through your mouth for seven seconds. This can be remarkably effective.

○ **Laugh.** Go to a live comedy show, see a funny film, or spend some time with children. This can often change your perspective.

○ **Sleep.** There are few things in life as healing as enough sleep. If you've been depriving yourself, revise your priorities to ensure a full eight hours each night.

○ **Cut out stimulants.** If you're drinking a lot of coffee or soda, switch to a beverage without caffeine.

○ **Help others.** Caring for other people in need—or even pets—might make you feel differently about your own troubles.

○ **Be physical.** Take a walk in the park...or better yet, a jog. Lift weights. Exercise. Any physical activity might help satisfy your body's "fight or flight" response.

Stress can be as debilitating as any disease. Don't let it damage your quality of life.

Embracing Exercise

It's been said that if exercise was a pill, every doctor would prescribe it. Exercise is a great antidote for stress. It can also help cure depression, anxiety, and many other ills.

Exercise strengthens every part of your body: your immune system, your hair and skin, your libido, your mind. In the past it was thought exercise could wear out joints. We now know that even the worst arthritis improves over time with exercise. Exercise can also increase energy and enthusiasm, and improve the quality of your sleep. Exercise lowers your risks for cancer, heart disease, diabetes, Alzheimer's, and stroke.

If you're perpetually tired and are chalking it up to old age, it might be that you're just not getting enough exercise. A 2010 study found that regular exercise can delay aging by as much as *12 years*.

If you haven't exercised for a while, go slow. Do a little, give yourself a day or two to recover, and then do a little more. The rest periods will provide your body the time it needs to adapt...and to build itself up for a healthier and happier new you.

The more care you take to avoid chemicals that mimic iodine, toxic chemicals overall, and toxic emotions such as stress, and the more effort you put into healing behaviors such as eating right and exercising, the more likely you are to overcome existing thyroid disorders, prevent the occurrence of new ones, and enjoy a vibrantly healthy life.

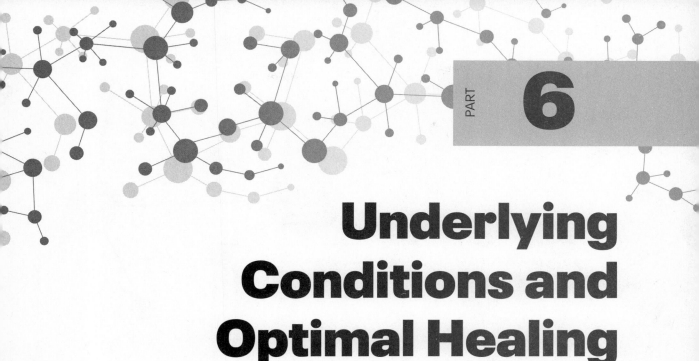

PART **6**

Underlying Conditions and Optimal Healing

In this last part, Chapter 21 identifies illnesses that frequently accompany thyroid disease—such as adrenal stress, diabetes, and heart disease—but are too often overlooked because they either have no obvious symptoms or have symptoms that are attributed to your already-diagnosed thyroid disease.

Finally, Chapter 22 shows you ways to identify a world-class thyroid physician and choose a top thyroid healthcare team.

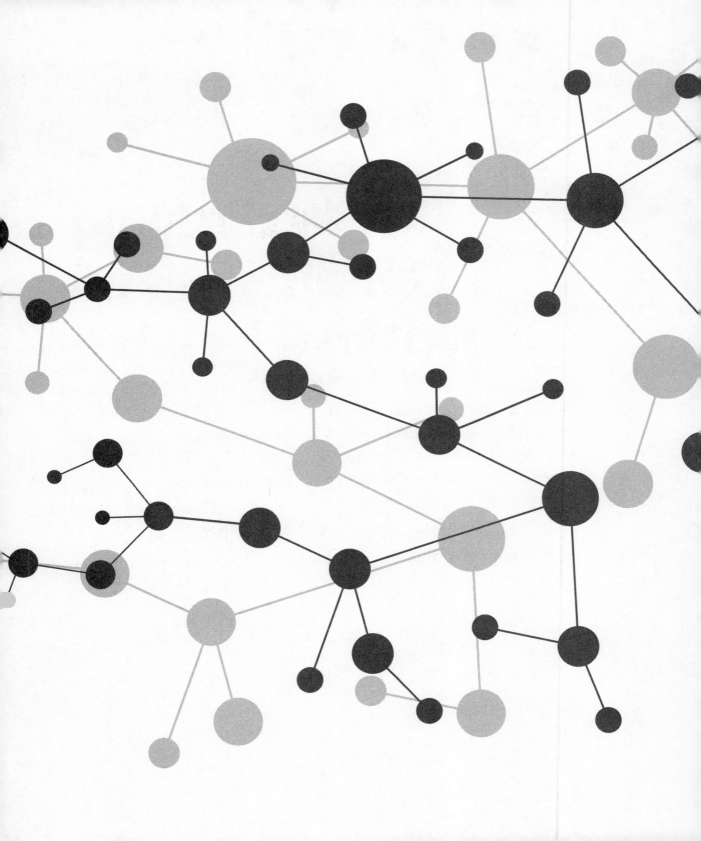

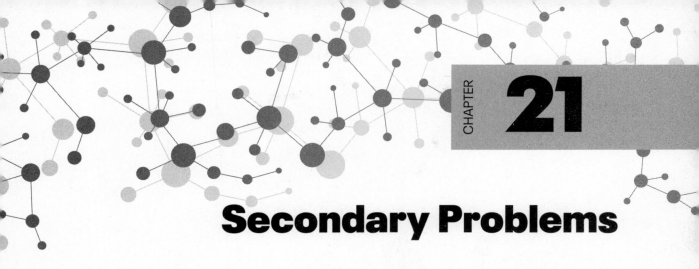

21

Secondary Problems

Imagine that you're already on the best thyroid medication and dosage for your condition, have tried all the strategies in Chapter 18...and after several months still don't feel well.

One possibility is that something's interfering with your medication. This can be remedied by taking your thyroid pill first thing in the morning with nothing but water, and waiting an hour before consuming anything else.

It could also be that something's changed since the last time you were tested. For example, your thyroid might have gotten either better or worse, making your current dosage out of sync with it. You can check on this by returning to your doctor for retesting.

However, it's also possible that you're doing everything right for your thyroid, but are suffering from one or more additional illnesses.

Each of the following diseases affect many people with thyroid disease:

- Adrenal stress
- Autoimmune gastritis
- Anemia
- Apnea
- Arthritis
- Celiac disease
- CFIDS
- Diabetes

    ○ Fatty liver disease

    ○ Fibromyalgia

    ○ H. Pylori

    ○ Heart disease

    ○ Kidney disease

    ○ Obesity

Of course, there are many other diseases that could potentially cause you problems. But in my experience, the ones on this list are the conditions that most often accompany thyroid disease and merit being kept in mind if you experience persistent symptoms your thyroid treatment doesn't appear to be addressing. This chapter provides the fundamentals you should know about each disease, covered in alphabetical order.

Adrenal Stress

Your adrenal glands produce scores of different types of hormones daily, regulating your blood sugar, blood electrolytes, wake and sleep cycles, fight or flight response, how well your cells absorb other hormones, and more.

It's very important that your adrenals produce their hormones, but it also matters *when* they produce them. For example, your adrenals normally make a burst of cortisol to wake you up and then gradually lower that level throughout the day. As cortisol drops off, your body gets the signal that it's time to slow down and sleep.

If you have adrenal stress, this cycle is thrown off balance. For example, you might find yourself waking up too early each morning, feeling fatigue in the afternoon, or getting sugar cravings each night.

Many doctors call this "adrenal fatigue." It's the wrong term, though, because the issue isn't that your adrenals are impaired or producing lower amounts of hormones. The problem is that their timing is off.

Chronic emotional stress is the most common cause for adrenal rhythms becoming disrupted. You're most at risk if you've had a high number of major stressors before age 18, such as abuse, neglect, a conflict between parents, or lack of emotional support.

Your doctor can check you for adrenal stress by testing your cortisol slope. This involves two salivary cortisol tests, one taken early in the morning and the other late at night. (Some versions of this testing go further by collecting four samples over the course of a day.) If you're healthy, your cortisol levels will be much higher in the morning than in the evening.

If the slope is abnormal, your doctor should perform further diagnostic tests to rule out any adrenal diseases (see Chapter 14).

Your past stressors can't be changed, but you can reduce or eliminate their negative effects by positive actions such as journaling, meditating, deepening your social connections, and helping other people.

It's also a good idea to cut out sugar and caffeine; spend time in sunlight in the morning; and maintain a consistent daily schedule for waking, eating, and going to sleep.

Anemia

Anemia refers to your blood failing to deliver enough oxygen throughout your body. This can happen if you've lost too much blood, aren't forming enough blood, or are making blood of insufficient quality to do its job properly. Typical symptoms include easily losing energy and feeling exhausted; a too-rapid heartbeat and shortness of breath from just moderate exertion; and difficulty concentrating.

This is a common condition. Studies have found that as many as 43 percent of patients with thyroid disease also have anemia.

You're most at risk if you're a menstruating women or have ongoing digestive issues. However, there are a wide range of potential causes, from the mild to the serious. So if you suspect you have anemia, have a doctor who's excellent at diagnosing diseases check you out.

Autoimmune Gastritis

Autoimmune gastritis (AIG) is a condition in which your immune system mistakenly attacks your stomach lining. This leads to chronic inflammation, and damage to the cells involved with absorbing nutrients such as vitamin B12, iron, folate, and zinc.

Symptoms may include frequent unexplained heartburn, gas, or bloating, as well as anemia resulting from key nutrients not being fully absorbed.

If symptoms persist, see your doctor and request she give you blood tests for parietal cell antibodies (PCA) and gastrin. If the results are positive, then an endoscope exam can check your stomach and esophagus for damage.

There's no formal medical treatment for AIG aside from giving you shots of vitamin B12, iron, folate, and/or zinc to compensate for the lack of absorption. However, try following the dietary suggestions in Chapter 18 to see if they help with both this condition and your thyroid.

Apnea

Sleep apnea is the inability to get enough oxygen throughout your body during sleep. When you're awake, breathing is easy because you're upright and have all your muscles working together. During the deepest stages of sleep, your diaphragm keeps working, but the many accessory muscles that help it stop responding to the signals from your brain (to prevent you from acting out your dreams).

Apnea can occur when your sinuses become congested or your jaw position shifts, which makes it harder for air to flow into your body. It can also happen if your brain fails to send the right signals to make your body breathe.

If you're a woman, you're three times more likely to have apnea than women without thyroid disease.

You won't be aware of apnea while it's happening. But clues include feeling your sleep hasn't been as deep and refreshing as you're used to; or someone sleeping with you telling you that you snore, breathe loudly through your mouth, and/or periodically hold your breath.

In many cases you can end this problem by simply sleeping on your side instead of on your back. Your tongue is less likely to obstruct your air passages when you're on your side.

You should also avoid alcohol before you go to bed, as it can hinder your brain's ability to control your breathing. Along the same lines, *don't* take sleep medication. If your air passages became obstructed and the medication kept you from being jarred awake, you might stop breathing.

If your nose is congested, then a nasal decongestant or nasal rinse might be all you need.

And if you have a weight issue, then shedding pounds will ease pressure on your diaphragm and might end the apnea. For a program to help you get thinner, see Chapter 19.

If none of these approaches help, then see a doctor who specializes in sleep disorders for additional solutions.

Arthritis

Arthritis is joint pain. Its symptoms are pain, stiffness, swelling, redness, and/or tenderness in one or more joints.

If the symptoms last for several days and occur multiple times per month, see a doctor. She'll probably give you a physical exam, x-rays, and blood tests. There are a number of different conditions that can cause arthritis, such as osteoarthritis and rheumatoid arthritis, and some are more treatable than others. A good diagnostician will hopefully narrow things down and then provide you with the right treatment.

One other approach worth trying is to follow the dietary suggestions in Chapter 18. If your pain decreases, then whatever is causing your thyroid disease is probably also causing your arthritis. In this case, stay on the diet. Over time, you might end up restoring your health from both conditions.

Celiac Disease

Celiac disease is an autoimmune disease that attacks your small intestine. It's triggered by gliadin, a protein found in wheat, barley, and rye. Symptoms can include digestive issues, diarrhea, gassiness, bloating, and poor absorption of nutrients. The latter can lead to fatigue, depression, rashes, numbness, and/or tingling.

Celiac disease can typically be detected with blood tests.

The treatment is to go on a strict and permanent gluten-free diet. In most cases, this will end the attacks on your small intestine and allow it to heal.

CFIDS

At some point you might have been diagnosed with chronic fatigue immunodeficiency syndrome (*CFIDS*), which results in ongoing fatigue so severe that it's debilitating. Other symptoms include insomnia, memory and concentration problems, weak muscles, and throat pain—all of which are also symptoms of thyroid disease.

As a "syndrome," CFIDS isn't so much a disease as a way of saying, "We don't know what's causing this." It's likely whatever is behind your thyroid disease is also behind your CFIDs.

If you've been treated by a doctor and are still experiencing these symptoms, first make sure you've been diagnosed correctly (see Chapter 7), and that you're on the thyroid medication and dosage most appropriate for you (see Chapters 8 and 9). In addition, consider trying both the dietary and antiviral/antibacterial supplements suggestions in Chapter 18 to see whether they make you feel better.

Diabetes

Diabetes is an abnormal elevation of blood sugar levels, primarily from an inability to make insulin (type 1) or a lack of response to insulin (type 2).

Thyroid disease patients are at increased risk for both types. However, by far the most common is type 2, with an estimated 30 million Americans suffering from it, so type 2 is what this section focuses on.

Symptoms of type 2 diabetes include frequent urination, increased thirst, continual hunger, fatigue, blurry vision, slow healing of cuts and wounds, patches of dark skin, itching, and yeast infections. But you can also have diabetes without any notable symptoms.

In addition to thyroid disease, factors that increase your risk of type 2 diabetes include a parent or sibling having it, excess weight, low levels of physical activity, high blood pressure (over 140/90), high LDL (bad) cholesterol, low HDL (good) cholesterol, high triglycerides, and getting older.

And for reasons we don't yet understand, you're also at increased risk if you're African American, Hispanic, Native American, Asian American, or a woman with polycystic ovary syndrome (PCOS).

The more risk factors you have, the more important it is that you make testing for diabetes a routine part of your annual checkup, even if you don't have any symptoms.

Typical tests include fasting blood sugar (checks your blood sugar level after you fast overnight) and hemoglobin a1c (determines the average amount of glucose in your blood over the last two to three months). If you have multiple risk factors, you should also consider an Insulin Fasting Test and a Glucose and Insulin Challenge Test.

A complication is that if you're hypothyroid, you can appear diabetic in lab results even when you're not. Be sure to see a doctor who understands this and will take it into account when interpreting your blood sugar levels.

In most cases, type 2 diabetes is reversible. One method for healing is a program I've developed called the Metabolism Reset Diet that's been used by thousands of diabetes patients. For details, see Chapter 19.

Fatty Liver Disease

The name *fatty liver disease* might sound funny, but it's a literal description. A healthy liver has about 1–3 percent fat. If that percentage grows to 10 percent or more, the excess fat gums up the liver and hinders it from functioning optimally.

Over time, fatty liver disease can lead to liver tissue scarring, liver cancer, and early death from liver damage. It also creates higher risk for diabetes and for heart disease (the most common cause of death for those with this condition).

Remember the song lyric, "Don't know what you've got 'til it's gone"? It's easy to not think about the numerous ways your liver keeps your body in balance—until it quits working.

Symptoms of fatty liver disease include excess weight; bloating, gas, or heartburn; reduced energy; muscles that don't repair as readily as they used to; and/or vague pain and discomfort in the upper-right portion of the abdomen. Because nerves are connected to each other in complex ways, sometimes patients also complain of pain in the right shoulder.

Studies have found as many as 30 percent of thyroid disease patients also have fatty liver disease. Other factors that make you more at risk of getting this condition include a genetic predisposition, type 2 diabetes (see previous section), excess weight, rapid weight loss, alcohol consumption, malnutrition, high cholesterol, high triglycerides, metabolic syndrome, and pregnancy.

Research indicates certain medications might also be risk factors, including aspirin, acetaminophen (Tylenol), steroids, tetracycline, tamoxifen, and calcium channel blockers (blood pressure pills such as diltiazem).

Fatty liver disease is most often diagnosed by an ALT (alanine aminotransferase) blood test, because when a liver is ailing it releases ALT into the bloodstream. An ALT level of 19 or higher for women, or 30 or higher for men, is suggestive of fatty liver disease. Be sure to get the precise number, because many labs set the top of their "normal" range higher than it should be, which can lead your doctor to conclude your liver is healthy when it really isn't.

Other diagnostic tools include physical exams, ultrasounds, and liver biopsies. It's a good idea to be checked for this condition annually.

Some experts predict fatty liver disease will become the top cause of liver transplants in the next decade, so it's a pressing healthcare issue.

The good news is it's also highly treatable.

To reverse fatty liver disease, you should entirely cut out alcohol. You should also lose excess weight (at a rate of 1–1.5 pounds per week, because rapid weight loss will make the condition worse); entirely cut out trans fatty acids (found in processed foods, baked goods, and animal fat); limit saturated fats; and manage your blood sugar.

Eating foods high in fiber and lean protein, and eating small frequent meals, can help heal your liver by balancing your blood sugar resistance. Fiber has a double benefit because it helps level your blood sugar, and it also binds with toxins that would otherwise go from your colon into your liver. Sources of high fiber include white beans, split peas, lentils, artichokes, broccoli, blackberries, and Brussels sprouts.

It's also good to consume magnesium, which acts as an antioxidant within the liver. Great sources of magnesium include adzuki beans, pumpkin seeds, avocados, and organic spinach.

Additionally helpful is vitamin E with mixed tocopherols, which you can buy as an over-the-counter supplement. Studies of liver biopsies have found vitamin E can halt the progression of fatty liver disease within five months.

Finally, consider following the program I've developed to help reverse fatty liver disease—as well as help you lose weight—called the Metabolism Reset Diet. For details, see Chapter 19.

Fibromyalgia

At some point you might have been diagnosed with fibromyalgia, a syndrome associated with ongoing pain in muscle tissues and chronic fatigue. However, those are also symptoms of thyroid disease; and as a "syndrome," fibromyalgia isn't so much a disease as a way of saying, "We don't know what's causing this." It's likely whatever is behind your thyroid disease is also behind your fibromyalgia.

If you've been treated by a doctor and are still experiencing these symptoms, first make sure you've been diagnosed correctly (see Chapter 7) and that you're on the thyroid medication and dosage most appropriate for you (see Chapters 8 and 9). In addition, consider trying both the dietary and antiviral/antibacterial supplements suggestions in Chapter 18 to see whether they make you feel better.

H. Pylori

H. pylori (helicobacter pylori) is a bacterium that lives in the stomach lining of an estimated 30–40 percent of Americans. Most people never get sick from it and so never realize they're hosting it. In more severe cases, though, it can lead to peptic ulcers (sores on your stomach lining or upper part of your small intestine), chronic stomach inflammation, and (rarely) stomach cancer.

Symptoms include acid reflux/heartburn and iron deficiency. If ulcers occur, you might feel a dull or burning pain in your stomach that comes and goes, especially between meals or at night. You might also experience bloating, burping, nausea, vomiting, loss of appetite, and mysterious weight loss.

H. pylori can also interfere with your absorption of thyroid medication. So if you need a higher dosage than someone at your weight normally would (see Chapter 9), that could indicate the bacterium's presence.

If you suspect you have H. pylori, you can try to combat it by consuming garlic, licorice root, broccoli sprouts, and green tea (which are all good for you regardless). You can also try both the dietary and antiviral/antibacterial supplements suggestions in Chapter 18.

Your doctor can check for H. pylori with a breath test, a blood test, a stool test, and/or a biopsy of the stomach done via endoscopy. The latter allows your doctor to identify the exact bacteria you have and prescribe the antibiotics most effective at killing it.

Heart Disease

Heart disease is the leading cause of death in the United States. That's partly because for one third of those with this condition, the first symptom of heart disease is a fatal heart attack. As a result, it's important that you get tested annually for any telltale signs of heart disease.

More than 47 percent of Americans have at least one of the three major risk factors for heart disease: high blood pressure, high cholesterol, and a history of smoking.

Untreated thyroid disease is a major risk factor, too. For example, if you have hypothyroidism, it can reduce your heart's ability to function and repair itself. And if you have hyperthyroidism, it can make your heart beat too rapidly, which has led to early deaths.

The problems hypothyroidism can create for the heart include:

O Decreased ability to pump blood

O Decreased function of the small arteries that regulate the flow of blood to tissues

○ Increased vascular resistance and diastolic blood pressure

○ Decreased flexibility of arteries

○ Atherosclerosis

○ Increased risk of coronary artery disease

These issues can decrease your heart's ability to work effectively by 30–50 percent.

The problems hyperthyroidism can create for the heart are even more severe. They include:

○ Increased heart rate

○ Atrial arrhythmia

○ Atrial fibrillation

○ Pulmonary hypertension

○ Left ventricular enlargement

○ Systolic hypertension

○ Wide pulse pressure

○ Ventricular arrhythmia

○ Low cardiac output

○ Heart failure

We therefore recommend that you be checked annually for heart disease via most or all of the following tests:

○ Blood pressure

○ Height to waist ratio

○ LDL cholesterol, a blood test that checks for bad cholesterol

○ Lipoprotein (a), another blood test that checks for bad cholesterol

○ Triglycerides, a blood test that checks for too high a level of fat

○ Fasting blood sugar, a blood test checking your sugar levels after you fast overnight

○ hs-CRP (high-sensitivity C-reactive protein), a blood test that measures inflammation

If any of these tests indicate you're at risk for heart disease, consider being evaluated by a cardiologist. This heart specialist will probably give you an exercise cardiac stress test in which you exercise on a stationary bike or treadmill while your heart is closely monitored.

Other things you can do to help ensure a healthy heart include eating well, lowering stress, and exercising. For more on these subjects, see Chapters 18 and 20.

If you take care to address all the issues that can harm your heart, you'll substantially increase your chances of living a long and vibrant life.

Kidney Disease

Chronic kidney disease, or *CKD*, is one of the top 10 causes of death in the United States, and it has a nasty synergy with thyroid disease.

You're at increased risk for CKD from hypothyroidism because a lowered metabolism can slow down your kidney's functioning; and from hyperthyroidism because a supercharged metabolism can dangerously speed the pace at which your kidney filters blood (called its glomerular filtration rate, or GFR).

At the same time, an impaired kidney will be less efficient at processing toxins and excess iodine out of your system, which could end up harming your thyroid. It'll also do a poorer job of helping to regulate the levels of T3 and T4 available to your cells.

This is an example of when lab ranges that are too broad can hurt you. If you have a TSH level of 2.85 or higher, research has found that it places you at increased risk for developing CKD, even though your level may be within the typical lab range of 0.4–4.5 mIU/L (see Chapter 7).

CKD is often overlooked because many of its symptoms are the same as those of thyroid disease. Common CKD symptoms include:

O Fatigue

O Fluid retention

O Brain fog

O Feeling cold

O Itchy skin

O Puffy eyes and face

Because it's so difficult to detect based on symptoms, your doctor should routinely give you urinalysis and blood tests for kidney disease as part of your annual checkup.

If it turns out you have CKD, treatment should focus on reducing or eliminating the factors that led to it. This includes managing your thyroid disease via medication and diet (see Chapters 8, 9, 12, and 18), and tightly regulating blood sugar, blood pressure, and blood cholesterol levels.

Obesity

Obesity is one of the most well-known symptoms associated with thyroid disease. What's less recognized is that the extra weight around and inside your organs can be a source of symptoms itself, including digestive issues, chronic fatigue, brain fog, depression, migraines, asthma, arthritis, and skin flare-ups.

Your percentage of excess organ fat can be inferred from your height-to-waist ratio. To determine this, measure your height in inches, and measure the circumference around your belly button in inches. Perform these measurements in the morning after you use the bathroom but before you eat anything. Then divide your waist circumference by your height.

For example, the calculation for a woman with a 32-inch waist who is 62 inches tall (5 feet 2 inches) would be as follows:

$$32 \div 62 = 51.6 \text{ percent}$$

To interpret your results, use this chart that shows the likelihood of your excess organ fat putting you at risk for health issues:

Ranges

	Extremely Slim	Healthy Slim	Healthy	Early risk	Significant risk	Severe risk
Women	<34%	35–41%	42–48%	49–53%	54–57%	>58%
Men	<34%	35–42%	43–52%	53–57%	58–62%	>63%

If you're at risk, consider following the weight loss program described in Chapter 19. It's specifically designed to reduce the fat around and inside your organs. If you can stick with it, you might experience a dramatic shrinkage of inches around your waist within the first few weeks.

As this chapter has shown, diagnosing precisely what's ailing you is a complex process. Ideally, you want a doctor who's superb at analyzing symptoms of thyroid disease and related diseases, knows the most appropriate tests to give you for any condition, and knows all the nuances involved in interpreting the results of those tests accurately. In addition, you want a doctor who makes use of all the information gathered to provide you with the best possible treatment. Ways you can identify such a doctor—including a list of questions you can ask to probe the physician's knowledge of thyroid disease—are covered in the next and final chapter.

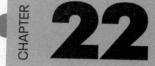

Choosing Optimal Thyroid Healthcare Providers

Chapter 4 described how to find the right doctor for you. This chapter goes a few steps further, explaining what types of doctors to avoid, why you might consider a team of healthcare providers, and questions you can ask to help identify a world-class thyroid physician.

Unhappy Patients

It's a sad fact that most thyroid patients are unhappy with the level of care they receive. It's typical for symptoms to go on for too long before thyroid disease is suspected; for testing to be incomplete; for lab results to be interpreted in less than optimal ways; and for a less than optimal medication to be prescribed. Too often, the result is treatment that fails to fully restore patient health.

In the 2018 survey described in Chapter 8, more than 12,000 people with thyroid disease were asked "How satisfied are you with the treatment you receive?", with the options ranging from 1 ("not satisfied") to 10 ("very satisfied"). Most of the respondents scored their treatment in the range of 1–4.

Responses to the question "How many times have you changed doctors because you were not satisfied with your thyroid treatment?" were also disheartening:

O 39 percent of respondents changed doctors 2–4 times

O 12 percent of respondents changed doctors 5–9 times

O 3 percent of respondents changed doctors more than 10 times

After treating thyroid disease for over two decades, I don't find these results at all surprising. A patient typically comes to see me because she's been trying to get help for years, but her local doctors failed her. The problem is usually a simple aspect of her care that was overlooked. Whenever I identify such an issue, I have conflicting feelings. Part of me is joyful that the patient will soon be feeling better. But another part of me is frustrated it took so long for her to find the care she needs and deserves.

Don't Let This Happen to You

Here's a composite story that represents the experiences of far too many of my patients while seeking medical help.

A woman in her mid-40s is suddenly struck with fatigue and depression, and gains unprecedented amounts of weight. Until this point, her relationship with her doctor has been fine. Most of her dealings with the medical world have been related to pregnancy, well-woman care, and the occasional bladder infection.

Her first point of medical distress occurs when the doctor tells her nothing is wrong. He explains her symptoms away with "You're just getting older." With a few casual words, her doctor is telling her to redefine her expectations for how well she should feel for the rest of her life—and that her new normal is to feel awful.

Not knowing any better, she accepts his prognosis and tries to live with the symptoms. However, they grow progressively worse. After a year of misery, a bunch of her hair falls out. She returns to the doctor and demands he take her more seriously. Her symptoms are so obvious at this point that even this doctor says, "You might have a thyroid issue. Let me see if we can confirm this with blood tests." She's relieved her doctor is finally acknowledging she has a legitimate medical problem, but is also deeply frustrated that she needlessly suffered for a year because he first assumed nothing was wrong.

The doctor receives her test results from the lab, finds that she is indeed hypo-thyroid, and prescribes synthetic T4. Unfortunately for her, she's among the third of the population who really needs a combination of T4 and T3. After several months on the medication, she's feeling only somewhat better. She's still fatigued, depressed, and gaining weight, and her hair is still falling out.

She finally gives up on her doctor and finds another one. But her new doctor has also been trained to prescribe only T4, so nothing changes.

Finally, she reaches out to my office in desperation. But at this point her attitude about all doctors is pretty dark.

Three Kinds of Doctors

When it comes to the thyroid, doctors tend to fall into three categories. The majority are committed to rigid protocols that often don't fully help. Typically, they'll test just TSH and free T4 (or even worse, just TSH), rely on lab-supplied ranges, never consider ordering an ultrasound, and prescribe only Synthroid or its generic equivalent levothyroxine.

At the other extreme, there are doctors happy to order any test you ask for and prescribe whatever you think is best. Their eagerness to be accommodating might seem positive, but it's based on their being more concerned with upsetting you than with jeopardizing your health.

The third category of doctors listen to you and pay careful attention to your symptoms, but also exercise the medical judgment they've developed from years of experience treating thousands of thyroid disease patients.

You should never ignore your feelings—or surrender your common sense—if a doctor seems to be dismissing your symptoms. At the same time, be wary of a doctor who reflexively agrees with anything you say. Try to find a physician who's going to work with you collaboratively while being committed to the best choices for your health.

Choosing an Optimal Team

Unraveling the symptoms of thyroid disease often takes a healthy relationship and orchestrated effort between you and your doctor. Beyond the basics of accurately diagnosing and testing for thyroid disease, ideally you'll work with a physician—or medical team—who understands three things:

○ The power of diet to correct thyroid disease

○ The importance of gently bringing your thyroid levels back to the optimal range for you—which includes knowing the nuances of how to interpret both test results and symptoms

O How to identify and treat other conditions that often exist alongside thyroid disease

One version of an effective team is the combination of a health coach and a prescriber who both understand the above.

The health coach can spend the most time with you, guiding you in how to eat and how to structure your life to help your recovery. The health coach can also give professional feedback to the prescriber about whether you appear to be doing well on your current thyroid hormone levels, whether you might be suffering from a secondary condition, and so on.

Meanwhile, the prescriber can help you understand your optimal thyroid hormone levels and guide you to them. She can help you reduce or end your thyroid medication if your body starts to work better on its own. She can also diagnose and effectively treat any secondary conditions that may be holding back your recovery.

A great healthcare provider will be a great communicator, making you feel that his top concern isn't his pet theory or his income, but your wellbeing. The best providers are those who connect with you and encourage you to achieve a level of health as good as, or better than, what you had before the thyroid diagnosis.

To locate doctors and other healthcare providers whose specialties include thyroid disease, use the "Finding Thyroid Healthcare Providers Near You" section in Appendix B.

Questions to Identify a World-Class Thyroid Doctor

The following are questions you can ask to help identify thyroid doctors and/or other thyroid healthcare providers who are among the best in the field.

You don't have to ask every question. You can simply pick out the ones that especially resonate with you.

You can ask these questions during your first appointment. In some cases, you might even be able to ask them by phone or email before committing to coming in.

How will you identify whether I have Hashimoto's versus some other hypothyroid disease? And does it even matter?

For Hashimoto's, which is an autoimmune disease, a doctor should test for a high level of thyroid peroxidase (TPO) antibodies and thyroglobulin (Tg) antibodies.

However, a negative result isn't definitive. If a patient has symptoms of Hashimoto's but the lab numbers don't confirm it, the doctor should prescribe an ultrasound performed directly on the thyroid to check for signs of cellular destruction.

Also, it *does* matter if you have Hashimoto's. Because it's an autoimmune disease, your doctor should check for signs of any related autoimmune disorders and any measurable stressors on your immune system.

Can you help my thyroid heal?

Virtually all physicians know that high overdoses of thyroid medication can do a lot of damage, and even shut down a thyroid permanently. However, not as many doctors realize that the right treatment can help a thyroid get better. A good doctor works hard to make sure your thyroid does as much as it can by itself.

What should I know about iodine?

Your thyroid needs iodine to function properly. However, iodine has become so prevalent in our diet over the past few decades that informed doctors are no longer worried about your getting too little. Instead, they worry about your taking in so much more than you need that it creates or exacerbates thyroid disease. A knowledgeable doctor will help you regulate your iodine intake to ensure the health of your thyroid.

Can you help me find the cause of my thyroid disease?

Most doctors assume nothing can be done to reverse hypothyroidism. The best doctors understand the disease can result from a variety of factors, including excess iodine, toxins, and infections. They'll work with you to discover your particular causes, and then try to safely stop those issues and give your thyroid the opportunity to heal.

What should I eat?

Most doctors believe diet has no role in thyroid treatment. Others latch onto the latest fad diet. The best doctors can help you choose the right foods to regulate iodine intake, guide you to a greater diversity of unprocessed natural foods, and more.

How do you feel about natural desiccated thyroid?

For most patients desiccated thyroid works at least as well, and often better, than synthetic thyroid medication. Because it contains T4, T3, T2, and T1, desiccated thyroid provides the most complete group of thyroid hormones of any medication.

Roughly one third of hypothyroid patients do poorly on T4-only synthetics and improve dramatically when switched to desiccated thyroid. Further, the converse isn't true—that is, patients on desiccated thyroid don't tend to improve by switching to T4-only medication.

Does my thyroid have any impact on my other hormones?

Thyroid hormones interact with every other hormone, including cortisol, estrogen, testosterone, melatonin, and DHEA. Most doctors don't take these interactions into account, and are surprised when a change in one upsets another. The best thyroid doctors keep all these hormones in mind. This is especially important for patients undergoing hormonal changes such as perimenopause or menopause.

Should I be screened for thyroid cancer?

In a word, yes. Thyroid cancer is one of the most rapidly increasing cancers in the United States, with over 50,000 cases a year. The best thyroid doctors screen all patients routinely and know how to adjust their care if nodules, calcifications, or other risk factors are found.

Does it matter what time of day I schedule for my blood tests?

If you have your blood taken at the wrong time of day—for example, too soon after taking your thyroid medication, or after taking certain supplements—the results can become meaningless. Most doctors fail to take these factors into account when interpreting test results. The best doctors advise their patients to schedule testing in the morning, and to not take any daily medications or supplements until after their blood has been drawn.

Is the normal range always best?

Many doctors pay no attention to findings within a lab's "normal" range. However, studies of people free of thyroid disease show their TSH and free T4 levels are in tighter ranges than the ones most labs use. The best thyroid physicians know this and interpret results using optimal ranges instead of lab-supplied ranges. These doctors also understand some patients might require even narrower ranges based on such factors as their ultrasound results.

Is it important to do follow-up blood tests?

Very. And yet patients typically have to reach out to their doctors to get retested. The best physicians know thyroid medication needs can change over time. They'll schedule you for testing multiple times your first year and then at least every six months afterward.

If my latest test results show I've become mildly hypothyroid but I'm still feeling fine, can I stick with my current dosage?

The dangers of thyroid disease go beyond the symptoms you feel. When not treated adequately, you're at higher risk for heart disease, some cancers, diabetes, and liver disease. The best doctors will adjust your medication to lower those risks, even when your symptoms appear to be well-controlled.

If my latest test results show my TSH is too low but I'm feeling fine, can I stick with my current dosage?

Some alternative doctors ignore low TSH, prescribing heavy-handed doses of thyroid medication. Most doctors realize that regardless of symptoms, too much thyroid medicine poses serious risks, including bone damage, brain damage, heart attacks, and early death.

When a patient overdosing on medication tells me he feels great, I respond, "You might feel great on cocaine, too. That doesn't mean it's good for you." The best doctors treat the causes of thyroid resistance for patients who seem to do well only on overdoses, so that these patients can feel at their best not only short term but sustainably for the rest of their lives.

We hope that this chapter, and this entire book, empowers you to obtain the finest testing, diagnosis, and treatment of whatever ails you.

And we wish you a life that's long, vibrant, joyful, and exceptionally healthy.

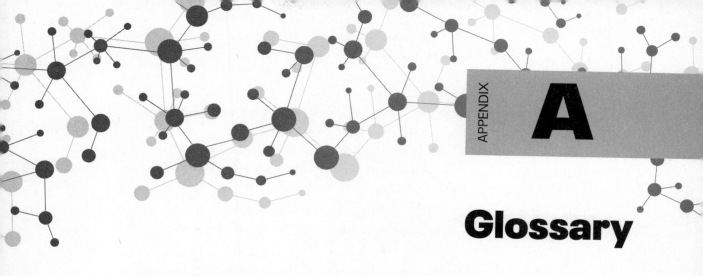

Glossary

Medical terms in this book are explained the first time they appear. If you're not reading the chapters in order, though, you might run across a term or acronym that's new to you. If this occurs, check this glossary for a brief definition. (And if you can't find the term here, also check the index.)

AACE   American Association of Clinical Endocrinologists (aace.com).

ACTH   Adrenocorticotropic hormone or corticotropin, which is made by your pituitary glands to regulate the hormone production of your adrenal glands.

Addison's disease   A physical problem with your adrenal glands (such as a genetic defect), or an autoimmune disorder in which they're being attacked by antibodies, that causes them to underperform. Also called adrenal insufficiency.

adenoma   A small non-cancerous growth.

adenosine triphosphate   See *ATP*.

adrenal glands   Two small triangle-shaped lumps of tissue residing over your kidneys that produce cortisol, which (among other things) helps convert T4 into T3, and allows T3 to enter cell membranes and access mitochondria.

adrenaline   A hormone produced by your adrenal glands in response to dangerous or unexpected situations. Adrenaline increases your heart rate, expands your blood vessels and air passages, and makes other subtle changes that help you react instantly by either battling or running (fight or flight).

adrenocorticotropic hormone   See *ACTH*.

alpha-lipoic acid   See *lipoic acid*.

antibodies Proteins used by your immune system to attack foreign invaders, such as bacteria and viruses. When your immune system mistakes your thyroid as a threat, it might attack those cells with thyroid peroxidase antibodies (TPO) and/ or thyroglobulin antibodies (Tg), resulting in Hashimoto's disease; or with thyroid stimulating immunoglobulin antibodies (TSI), resulting in Graves' disease.

antithyroid medications Drugs such as Tapazole/methimazole and propylthiouracil (PTU) that manage hyperthyroidism by interfering with your thyroid's ability to make its hormones.

Armour Thyroid Medication made from desiccated pig thyroid that contains all four thyroid hormones: T4, T3, T2, and T1. Manufactured by Allergan (ArmourThyroid.com).

atenolol A beta blocker that's effective at slowing a rapid heartbeat caused by hyperthyroidism.

ATP Adenosine triphosphate, the energy created from the conversion of glucose by the mitochondria in your cells.

autoimmune disease A condition in which your immune system mistakenly attacks an area of your body. More than 80 percent of thyroid disease cases are caused by Hashimoto's (hypothyroidism) and Graves' (hyperthyroidism), both of which the medical community believes attack your thyroid with antibodies.

basal temperature tests An old-fashioned test used to identify hypothyroidism via body temperature. It's been made obsolete by modern lab tests, which are much more reliable and precise.

beta blocker A medication that blocks the effects of adrenaline, making your heart beat more slowly and with less force. It also helps reduce your blood pressure and improve your blood's circulation. The best beta blockers for hyperthyroidism include atenolol and propranolol.

biopsy See *fine needle aspiration biopsy* and *coarse needle biopsy*.

block-and-replace therapy A technique for managing hyperthyroidism in which your doctor blocks the disease with antithyroid medication while simultaneously replacing any lack of hormones with thyroid medication.

Brazil nut Your best source of selenium. Eat just one a day because consuming more than that risks an eventual selenium overdose.

bromocriptine   A medication used to slow the growth of, and often shrink, an adenoma on the pituitary gland.

cancer   See *thyroid cancer*.

cholecystokinin   A hormone that stimulates the digestion of fat and suppresses hunger. One reason to eat a moderate amount of healthy fat every meal is to produce this hormone, which effectively tells your brain that you're full and so makes you less likely to overeat.

coarse needle biopsy   A procedure for a potentially cancerous nodule three quarters of an inch or larger; it employs a needle to extract tissue samples for examination in a lab. See also *fine needle aspiration biopsy*.

cold nodule   See *thyroid nodule*.

compounded thyroid medication   Thyroid medication prepared by a compounding pharmacy instead of a drug manufacturer (which has greater quality assurance and post-production analysis). It's normally fine to use a compounding pharmacy, but thyroid hormones are so minute that the risk of a mistake being made outweighs any convenience gained by compounding.

comprehensive metabolic panel (CMP)   A very common test that identifies the levels of a variety of critical chemicals in your bloodstream, including calcium (which is useful if you suspect a problem with your parathyroid glands). Also called a chemistry panel, chemistry screen, and SMAC test.

conjugated linoleic acid (CLA)   A natural dietary supplement that can help combat *insulin resistance* by re-sensitizing insulin cell receptors. See also *lipoic acid*.

corticotropin   See *ACTH*.

cortisol   A critical hormone produced by your adrenal glands. Its many functions include regulating your blood's glucose levels, controlling your blood pressure, healing inflammation, helping convert T4 into T3, and allowing T3 to enter cell membranes and access mitochondria.

cortisol challenge test   A test in which you're given a small dose of ACTH to see how much cortisol your adrenal glands produce in response, which provides precise information on your adrenals' health. See also *salivary cortisol testing*.

Cushing's syndrome A condition in which weight gain, weakened immunity, thinning skin and hair, and other problems are caused by too much cortisol. See also *pheochromocytoma*.

Cytomel Thyroid medication that's a synthetic version of T3, manufactured by Pfizer (Pfizer.com). The generic version is liothyronine.

cytopathologist A doctor who's an expert at analyzing cells extracted via a biopsy.

deiodinase type 1 The enzyme your body uses to strip off an iodine atom from a thyroid hormone molecule and convert it into a different hormone—most notably, turning T4 into T3. See also *selenium*.

desiccated thyroid Medication made from desiccated pig thyroid that contains all four thyroid hormones: T4, T3, T2, and T1. Also called glandular thyroid, natural desiccated thyroid, or NDT. Brand name versions of this medication include Armour Thyroid, Nature-Throid, and WP Thyroid.

desiccated thyroid powder The raw material used to make desiccated thyroid, manufactured by American Laboratories (AmericanLaboratories.com).

do-iodothyronine See *T2*.

endocrine system A group of glands that secrete hormones regulating how your body functions. The glands include the thyroid, parathyroids, pancreas, ovaries, testes, adrenals, pineal, pituitary, and hypothalamus.

endocrinologist A doctor who specializes in disorders of the glands of the endocrine system and their hormones.

ENT Ear, nose, and throat surgeon, which is typically the doctor needed for thyroid cancer.

eye disease See *hyperthyroid eye disease*.

fine needle aspiration biopsy A procedure that employs a very thin needle to extract tissue samples from any potentially cancerous nodules on your thyroid for examination in a lab. See also *coarse needle biopsy*.

fluoride A mineral primarily used for dental health that can interfere with your thyroid's production of hormones. Fluoride can cause or worsen hypothyroidism, but is an inexpensive and relatively harmless remedy for hyperthyroidism (either by itself or combined with medication such as Tapazole).

follicular thyroid cancer   The second most common form of thyroid cancer, accounting for about 12 percent of cases. Its cure rate is 97 percent. See also *thyroid cancer.*

free T3   The amount of T3 in your bloodstream that's available for powering up your cells (as opposed to the T3 that's rendered inert by being bound by proteins). Measuring free T3 is one of the ways to determine your thyroid's status.

free T4   The amount of T4 in your bloodstream that's available for conversion to T3 (as opposed to the T4 that's rendered inert by being bound by proteins). Measuring free T4 is one of the ways to determine your thyroid's status.

glandular thyroid   See *desiccated thyroid.*

glucose   A fundamental sugar your body creates from the food you eat. The mitochondria in your cells convert it into energy.

goiter   A large non-cancerous growth on your thyroid, which typically results from a lack of iodine or hyperthyroidism.

Graves' disease   An autoimmune disease in which your immune system mistakes your thyroid for a threat and attacks it with TSI antibodies. More than 80 percent of hyperthyroidism cases are caused by Graves' disease.

Hashimoto's disease   An autoimmune disease in which your immune system mistakes your thyroid for a threat and attacks it with antibodies. Roughly 75–85 percent of hypothyroidism cases are caused by Hashimoto's disease.

Hashitoxicosis   A manifestation of Hashimoto's disease that swings you back and forth between hyperthyroidism (during antibody attacks that slaughter thyroid cells, spilling out their stored hormones) and hypothyroidism (between attacks, as the thyroid becomes increasingly less functional). These extreme states can average out, making your TSH appear normal.

hot nodule   See *thyroid nodule.*

hyperthyroid eye disease   Ocular problems from hyperthyroidism, and especially Graves' disease, including "lid lag" (see Chapter 10), sensitivity to light, feeling painful dryness or grittiness in the eyes, double vision, and eyelids retracting while the eyes enlarge and protrude to create a "bug-eyed" look.

hyperthyroidism   A disease that causes your thyroid to produce too much of its hormones, leading to dangerous overstimulation of your body's cells. Common symptoms include a pounding heart, anxiety, panic attacks, tremors, and goiters.

hypothalamus   The portion of your brain that (among other things) senses when your body needs more energy and sends a chemical signal to your pituitary gland to make more TSH.

hypothyroidism   A disease in which you don't have enough thyroid hormones to provide your body's cells with the energy they need. Common symptoms include fatigue, weight gain, depression, slowed thinking, and hair loss. Experts estimate 1 in 10 Americans suffers from hypothyroidism.

insulin resistance   A condition in which your cell receptors designed to respond to insulin become less sensitive, requiring your body to pump out significantly more insulin than normal. This can lead to decreased fat burning, increased inflammation, and diseases such as high blood pressure. You can potentially resensitize the cell receptors by taking *conjugated linoleic acid (CLA)* and/or *lipoic acid*.

iodine   The element your thyroid combines with tyrosine to make its hormones.

iodine uptake and thyroid scan   Test that involves injecting you with or having you swallow a tiny amount of radioactive iodine, waiting 6–24 hours, and then scanning your neck to get a clear picture of what's happening in your thyroid.

iodine-induced thyroiditis   See *thyroiditis*.

isthmus   The middle section of your thyroid, connecting its left and right lobes.

IU/mL   International unit for antibodies per milliliter of blood, used to measure TPO and Tg antibodies.

kava-kava   A natural remedy that may help calm anxiety due to hyperthyroidism. See also *theanine*.

lean body mass (LBM)   The parts of your body that are fat-free, including your muscles and bones.

levothyroxine   Thyroid medication that's a generic synthetic version of T4. The most prescribed brand name version is Synthroid.

Levoxyl   Thyroid medication that's a synthetic version of T4, manufactured by Pfizer (Levoxyl.com). The generic version is levothyroxine.

liothyronine   Thyroid medication that's a synthetic version of T3. The brand name version is Cytomel.

lipoic acid   A natural dietary supplement that can help combat *insulin resistance* by re-sensitizing insulin cell receptors. See also *conjugated linoleic acid (CLA)*.

lobes   The left and right parts of your thyroid gland. If one lobe fails or is removed, the other can take over the job of making hormones.

magnesium   A natural remedy for a rapid heartbeat caused by hyperthyroidism.

mcg   Short for microgram.

medullary thyroid cancer   The third most common form of thyroid cancer, accounting for about 5 percent of cases. The recommended treatment is surgically removing the entire thyroid, possibly the lymph nodes, and anywhere else it appears to have invaded.

MEN1 syndrome   Multiple endocrine neoplasia 1, a rare condition in which several different endocrine glands—the thyroid, parathyroids, pancreas, pituitary, and/or adrenals—start growing tumors at the same time. These tumors usually aren't cancerous, but they lead to an overproduction of hormones. Also known as Werner's syndrome.

MEN2 syndrome   Multiple endocrine neoplasia 2, a rare condition in which various endocrine glands start growing cancerous tumors at the same time. Also known as Sipple's syndrome.

metabolism   Your body's energy level, which is set by your hypothalamus and enforced by your thyroid's hormones.

methimazole   Medication that very effectively combats even severe hyperthyroidism by interfering with the thyroid's ability to make its hormones. The brand name version is Tapazole.

mg   Short for milligram. Equivalent to 1,000 mcg.

mitochondria   The "power plants" in each of your cells that take glucose and convert it into energy, or ATP.

mIU/L   Milli-international units per liter of blood, used to measure TSH.

mono-iodothyronine   See *T1*.

multiple endocrine neoplasia 1 See *MEN1 syndrome.*

multiple endocrine neoplasia 2 See *MEN2 syndrome.*

natural desiccated thyroid See *desiccated thyroid.*

Nature-Throid Medication made from desiccated pig thyroid that contains all four thyroid hormones: T4, T3, T2, and T1. Manufactured by RLC Labs (RLCLabs. com). This medication is identical to RLC's WP Thyroid.

NDT See *desiccated thyroid.*

ng/dL Nanograms per deciliter of blood, used to measure free T4.

nodule See *thyroid nodule.*

painful subacute thyroiditis See *thyroiditis.*

papillary thyroid cancer The most common form of thyroid cancer, accounting for about 80 percent of cases. It's typically caused by exposure to radiation. Its cure rate is 97 percent. See also *thyroid cancer.*

parathyroid glands Small glands residing behind your thyroid that regulate the amount of calcium in your blood and bones.

pg/dL Picograms per deciliter of blood, used to measure free T3.

pheochromocytoma A condition in which your adrenal glands' cells spawn tumors that grow either on the glands or outside of them, and produce hormones independently, resulting in too much cortisol. See also *Cushing's syndrome.*

pituitary disease Underactivity or overactivity of the pituitary gland most caused by one or more tumors. If a pituitary tumor is 14 millimeters or smaller, it can usually be shrunk with the medicine bromocriptine. Otherwise, surgery is required.

pituitary gland A pea-size organ just above your sinuses that, among other things, regulates the hormone production of your thyroid (via TSH) and adrenal glands (via ACTH).

Plummer's disease The second most common cause of hyperthyroidism, resulting in one or more non-cancerous nodules that produce hormones independently— without waiting to be stimulated by TSH. Also called Plummer's adenoma (when there's just one nodule) or toxic multinodular goiter.

postpartum thyroiditis See *thyroiditis.*

propranolol   A beta blocker that's effective at slowing a rapid heartbeat caused by hyperthyroidism.

PTU (propylthiouracil)   Medication that combats hyperthyroidism by interfering with the thyroid's ability to make its hormones. PTU has largely been replaced by the superior medication Tapazole but is useful if you're allergic to Tapazole, find Tapazole ineffective, or are pregnant.

radioiodine ablation   A procedure designed to end hyperthyroidism via radioactive iodine that destroys a substantial percentage of the thyroid's cells, making it too small to continue overproducing hormones. This procedure is also used to destroy remaining thyroid cells after the thyroid is removed (typically due to cancer).

red blood cell element test   Measures your three-month average levels of essential chemicals boron, chromium, calcium, copper, iron, magnesium, manganese, molybdenum, phosphorus, potassium, selenium, vanadium, and zinc; and detects the presence of the toxins arsenic, cadmium, lead, mercury, and thallium.

resting metabolic rate (RMR)   A measure of your base level of activity (your heart beating, your lungs breathing, your brain processing information, and so on) when you're not doing anything strenuous.

reverse T3   A nonfunctional thyroid hormone your body creates by removing an iodine atom from obsolete or excess T4. The resulting reverse T3 can then be easily flushed from your system.

RMR   See *resting metabolic rate*.

salivary cortisol testing   A test in which you take a sample of your saliva periodically over 24 hours, which allows your doctor to track your cortisol levels throughout the day. See also *cortisol challenge test*.

selenium   The chemical your body uses to make the enzyme deiodinase type 1 effective. You can ensure you have enough selenium by eating a single Brazil nut a day. (Don't eat more than one a day regularly, though, or you could end up overdosing.)

shoulder stand   Yoga posture in which you lie flat on your back, letting your body rest on your shoulders and the back of your neck, and raise your legs together until they're pointing straight up. This places substantial compression on your thyroid and can increase the blood supply to it.

silent thyroiditis   See *thyroiditis.*

Sipple's syndrome   See *MEN2 syndrome.*

struma ovarii   A rare condition in which thyroid cells grow in the ovaries. If these cells produce hormones independently, they'll make you hyperthyroid. They're treated via surgical removal.

Synthroid   Bestselling thyroid medication that's a synthetic version of T4, manufactured by Abbott (Abbott.com). The generic version is levothyroxine.

T1   A thyroid hormone with one iodine atom. No useful function has been discovered for T1 so far, but that might change with further research. Also called mono-iodothyronine.

T2   A thyroid hormone with two iodine atoms that studies have found plays a role in metabolism and burning fat. Also called do-iodothyronine.

T3   A thyroid hormone with three iodine atoms that does the work of powering up the mitochondria in your cells. Also called triiodothyronine. Taking T3 medication can be especially effective in lifting depression.

T4   A thyroid hormone with four iodine atoms designed to circulate in your bloodstream, and be stored in your tissues, until it's needed to be converted into T3. Also called thyroxine or tetra-iodothyronine.

Tapazole   Medication that very effectively combats even severe hyperthyroidism by interfering with the thyroid's ability to make its hormones. The generic version is methimazole.

tetra-iodothyronine   See *T4.*

Tg   Thyroglobulin antibodies, which attack your thyroid and cause the autoimmune disease Hashimoto's.

theanine   A natural remedy which might help calm anxiety caused by hyperthyroidism. See also *kava-kava.*

thyroglobulin   The protein your thyroid binds with iodine to make its hormones.

thyroglobulin antibodies   See *Tg.*

thyroid   A butterfly-shaped gland that resides in your neck. It produces T4, T3, T2, and T1 hormones that regulate the energy level, growth, and reproduction of every cell in your body.

thyroid cancer   A serious but seldom fatal disease that's typically treated with surgery and radioactive iodine. The most common forms are papillary and follicular, which have a cure rate of 97 percent.

thyroid disease   A medical condition of your thyroid, such as hypothyroidism, hyperthyroidism, or thyroid cancer.

thyroid eye disease   See *hyperthyroid eye disease.*

thyroid nodule   A small growth on your thyroid. If a scan indicates the nodule is "cold," meaning it's not absorbing iodine and or making hormones, there's about a 10 percent chance it's cancerous. Alternatively, if the nodule is "hot," it's producing hormones and may be making you hyperthyroid.

thyroid peroxidase antibodies   See *TPO.*

thyroid scan   See *iodine uptake* and *thyroid scan.*

thyroid stimulating hormone   See *TSH.*

thyroid stimulating immunoglobulin   See *TSI.*

thyroid storm   A condition in which you're so overloaded with thyroid hormones that you're at risk of a heart attack. The quickest way to end this condition is to overload your thyroid with iodine, which "blows a fuse" and temporarily shuts down your thyroid.

thyroiditis   A condition in which antibodies attack and inflame your thyroid. This usually stems from Hashitoxicosis, but can also result from (typically) temporary illnesses such as painful subacute thyroiditis (triggered by a respiratory infection), silent thyroiditis (which causes no pain), postpartum thyroiditis (which occurs after pregnancy), and iodine-induced thyroiditis (which is caused by iodine overdosing).

thyrotoxicosis factitia   A condition in which hyperthyroidism occurs as a result of artificial rather than natural causes, such as an overdose of thyroid medication.

thyroxine   See *T4.*

total T3   The total amount of T3 in your body—that is, both free T3 and the T3 bound by proteins. This information seldom has practical value, as what matters is free T3.

total T4   The total amount of T4 in your body—that is, both free T4 and the T4 bound by proteins. This information seldom has practical value, as what matters is free T4.

toxic nodule   A small non-cancerous growth that produces thyroid hormones independently. This is a result of Plummer's disease.

TPO   Thyroid peroxidase antibodies, which attack your thyroid and cause the autoimmune disease Hashimoto's.

triiodothyronine   See *T3*.

TSH   Thyroid stimulating hormone, made by your pituitary gland to instruct your thyroid gland to increase its T4, T3, T2, and T1 production. Measuring your TSH level (which is a 2–3 month average) is one of the ways to determine your thyroid's status.

TSH-secreting pituitary adenoma   See *pituitary disease.*

TSI   Thyroid stimulating immunoglobulin, which are antibodies that attack your thyroid and cause the autoimmune disease Graves'.

tyrosine   The amino acid that your thyroid combines with iodine to make its hormones.

ultrasound   Safe and inexpensive test that can create images of your thyroid by bouncing high-frequency sound waves off it.

Unithroid   Thyroid medication that's a synthetic version of T4, manufactured by Amneal Pharmaceuticals (Unithroid.com). The generic version is levothyroxine.

Werner's syndrome   See *MEN1 syndrome.*

WP Thyroid   Medication made from desiccated pig thyroid that contains all four thyroid hormones: T4, T3, T2, and T1. Manufactured by RLC Labs (RLCLabs.com). This medication is identical to RLC's Nature-Throid.

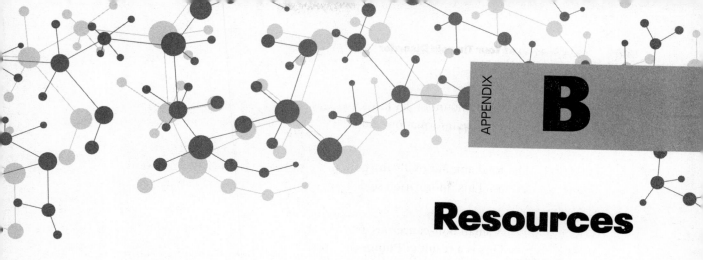

Resources

There are organizations and websites available to help you locate the right doctor, learn more about thyroid disease, and research thyroid medications. This appendix describes some of the very best of these information sources.

Finding Thyroid Healthcare Providers Near You

Finding a thyroid doctor who's highly skilled, and yet willing to collaborate with you on your diagnosis and treatment, isn't always easy. Neither is finding other thyroid healthcare providers, such as nutritionists who can help you maintain a thyroid-friendly diet. The following organizations and websites will help.

In addition, see Chapters 4 and 22, which explain what to seek and what to avoid in a thyroid healthcare provider.

American Association of Naturopathic Physicians
Web: Naturopathic.org

This professional organization consists of alternative health practitioners who "teach their patients to use diet, exercise, lifestyle changes, and cutting-edge natural therapies to enhance their bodies' ability to ward off and combat disease," and who "blend the best of modern medical science and traditional natural medical approaches to not only treat disease but also restore health." If you want to feel assured that your request for desiccated thyroid won't lead to a confrontation with your doctor, click this site's "Find an ND" button to search by location, telemedicine availability, and/or specialty (choose the "Endocrinology" option).

Endocrine Association of Naturopathic Physicians
Web: EndoANP.org/find-an-nd

The Endocrine Association of Naturopathic Physicians is a group of naturopathic doctors who focus on endocrinology, including thyroid care. You can use the web page above to find members in your area.

American Association of Clinical Endocrinologists
Web: AACE.com/find-an-endo

The American Association of Clinical Endocrinologists consists of endocrinologists, primary care physicians, and other health care professionals who treat patients with endocrine conditions, including thyroid disease. You can use the web page above to find members in your area by entering your zip code and how large an area you want to search, and then choosing to display the results as either a list or a map.

American Thyroid Association
Web: Thyroid.org/patient-thyroid-information/endocrinology-thyroid-doctor

The American Thyroid Association is a medical society consisting of more than 1,700 thyroid healthcare providers. You can use the web page above to find pertinent members in your area by selecting your state, clicking the "Disorder" option, and then selecting the thyroid issue for which you want help (for example, *Hypothyroidism, Hyperthyroidism,* or *Thyroid Cancer*).

Thyroid Top Doctors
Web: Thyroid-info.com/topdrs/#us

Author and thyroid patient advocate Mary Shomon runs this site that lists U.S. thyroid doctors nominated by patients. According to Shomon, a top physician is "a doctor who listens, cares, has an open mind, wants us to understand and participate in our treatment decisions, and isn't beholden to a particular drug company." Included are endocrinologists, thyroid specialists, thyroid surgeons, integrative physicians, and more. First click on your state, then scroll through the list to find doctors in your city.

American Board of Medical Specialties
Web: CertificationMatters.org

If you want to check whether a U.S. doctor you're considering is board certified in his or her specialty, click this site's "Is My Doctor Certified?" button, then specify your doctor by first name, last name, state, and/or specialty.

Integrative Health Care
Web: IntegrativeHealthCare.com

If you'd like to be helped by the health center founded by the co-author of this book, the doctors at Integrative Health are all personally guided by Dr. Alan Christianson, focus solely on thyroid disease, and are trained in both conventional medicine and diet/lifestyle therapies. You can work with them using telemedicine from any state in America.

Learning More About Thyroid Disease

We've tried to cover everything you're likely to need to know about thyroid disease in this book, but there might be times when you require additional information. You can use the following websites to fill in further details and/or breaking news.

Thyroid Disease Manager
Web: ThyroidManager.org

This excellent site is written by doctors and for doctors. It's quite technical, so if jargon makes you uncomfortable, steer clear. Otherwise, you can find a wealth of information here focused directly on thyroid disease.

PubMed
Web: PubMed.ncbi.nlm.nih.gov

The U.S. Government's National Institutes of Health run this invaluable site, which is a clearinghouse for virtually all published medical research—including studies of thyroid disease. The material is as technical as it gets, but if you need to perform cutting-edge research, this is the place to start.

Medline Plus
Web: MedlinePlus.gov

The U.S. Government's National Institutes of Health also run this site, which—in contrast to PubMed—is designed to be patient friendly. It provides a great deal of solid information about all major illnesses, including thyroid disease.

Thyroid Cancer Survivors' Association
Web: thyca.org

Information about both thyroid cancer and support groups for those struck by the disease can be found at this site run by thyroid cancer survivors since 1995.

Thyroid Medication Manufacturers

If you're trying to decide which thyroid medications to choose (as discussed in Chapters 3 and 8), you might find it useful to explore the websites of their manufacturers. They are as follows:

Synthroid (Abbott)
Web: Abbott.com

Cytomel and Levoxyl (Pfizer)
Web: Pfizer.com and Levoxyl.com

Unithroid (Amneal Pharmaceuticals)
Web: Unithroid.com

Nature-Throid and WP Thyroid (RLC Labs)
Web: RLCLabs.com

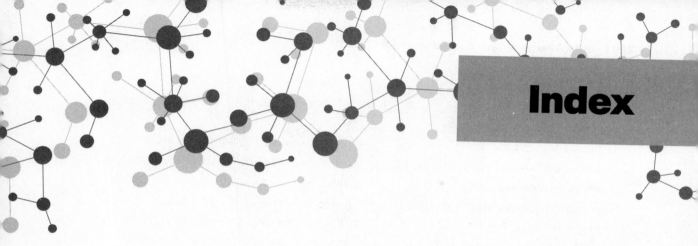

Index